MILLIE, M.D.

For Eleanor —

3/27/99

Read and enjoy !

Helen Strayer

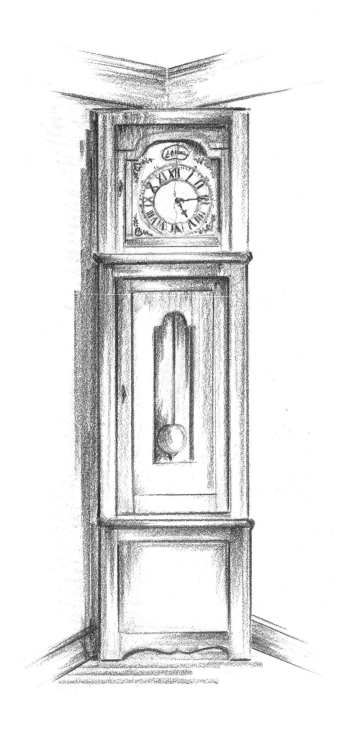

MILLIE, M.D.

The Story of a Nineteenth Century Woman

1846 - 1927

HELEN DANN STRINGER

North Country Books, Inc.
Utica, New York

MILLIE, M.D.
The Story of a Nineteenth Century Woman
1846-1927

Copyright © 1992
by
Helen Dann Stringer

ISBN 0-925168-07-6

Library of Congress Cataloging-in-Publication Data

Stringer, Helen Dann, 1909-
    Millie M.D.: the story of a nineteenth century
woman, 1846-1927 / by Helen Dann Stringer.
        p.   cm.
    ISBN 0-925168-07-6
    1. DeMott, Amelia Dann, 1846-1927.   2.
Women physicians — New York (State) — Biography.
I. Title.
R154.D44S87   1992
610'.92 — dc20
(B)   92-38434
                                             CIP

Published by
North Country Books, Inc.
18 Irving Place
Utica, New York 13501

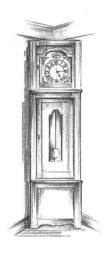

A GREAT-GREAT-GREAT GRANDFATHER'S CLOCK
1817-1992

This story of Millie, M.D. is dedicated to a clock that belonged to her during her lifetime — although it existed before she was born and after her death. The heartbeat of the clock has sounded throughout the successive lives of related men, women and children for one hundred seventy-five years.

Its pulse has persisted strong and regular. Its chime has cheered those who have lived in intimate association with it through times of birth and death, through times of war and peace, through times of adversity and prosperity. Its unremitting marking off of hours and minutes has persisted day and night as the swinging pendulum accompanied a familiar deep-toned sound.

The clock, in spite of its inanimate character, has become over the years a spiritual symbol — a symbol of one long life well-lived — the life of Millie, M.D.

CONTENTS

ACKNOWLEDGMENTS

I extend gratitude to friends far and near for their patience as the pace of my life has shifted during the past few years to energy-conserving apportionment of time. With deep affection I am grateful to my sons, Dann, Dick, David, Chris and Andy for their continuous support and understanding, and to my daughter, Nancy, for her tender insights and creative curiosity concerning her Great-grandmother—the woman doctor who lived so long ago, to my grandson Douglas for his technical ability to calm my "Macintosh frustrations" and to my grandson Micah for his fine drawing of the great-grandfather clock. To all of you I say thank you.

With heartfelt appreciation I recognize my editor, Cynthia Maude-Gembler, for her wise, untiring, good-natured assistance in the preparation of this book for publication.

In addition I extend gratitude to the staff and co-participants of the Vermont Breadloaf Writers' Conference of 1988, especially to mentors, Ron Powers and David Bain.

> Helen D. Stringer
> Manlius, NY
> September, 1992

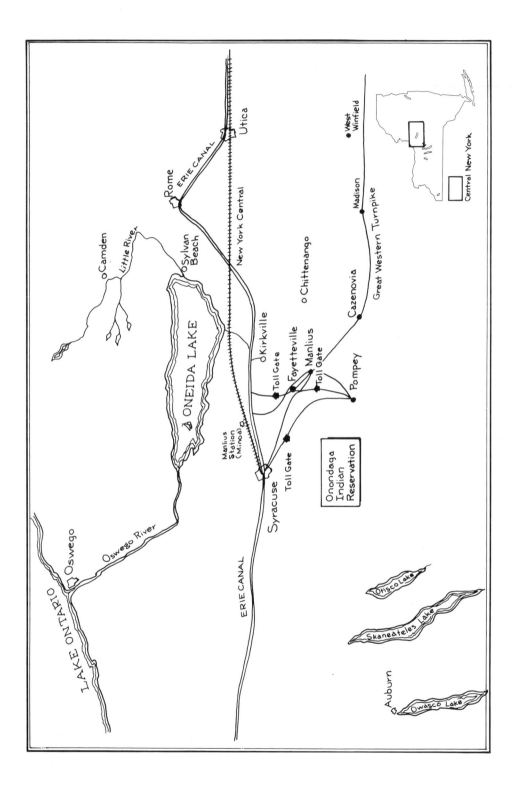

PREFACE

My Grandmother, known in the city of Syracuse as Millie, M.D., was a practicing physician from 1878 to 1905. As a doctor, she devoted herself chiefly to women — providing care during illness and life crises. Disease prevention and public health were her interests. She became a teacher of hygiene and good nutrition to wives and mothers as care-givers themselves.

During the last twenty years of her life, my paternal Grandmother — Amelia Dann DeMott — occupied the large red brick house across the driveway from our family home in upstate New York. With my Grandfather, she welcomed me and my four brothers and sisters at any hour of the day or night. Their doors were unlocked: their arms open.

When I was nine years old, our Mother died from a massive hemorrhage at the birth of the fifth child. The relationship between my Grandmother and me grew closer year by year.

Toward the end of her life my Grandmother entrusted me with a collection of her letters, papers and early photographs. While I treasured the possession, it was not until recently that I realized I was the only person who could write the detailed story of my Grandmother's life. As an octogenarian myself, I began to piece together portions of letters and documents, call up memories from long ago, filter through archives and family tintype pictures — even becoming computer-literate myself for the task of writing Millie's story.

My purpose in pursuing the challenge has been to preserve the unusual account of a young woman facing disease, early widowhood, single parenthood, and discrimination both as a medical student and later as a practicing woman physician. Endowed with high energy and dedication to her profession, she became a force in her community as a supporter of women's rights, a compassionate doctor, and a caring mother.

Beyond the limits of a family chronicle, Millie's story deserves a hearing. Her voice represents the voices of many women—those who over the years have served in the fields of medicine, public health, and human understanding—those whose voices have since been silenced.

This story is written in the form of a characterization of the times and challenges my Grandmother faced. Unlike a scholarly biography, the formulation of this story has depended on interpretation of family life and on deep searching of my own memory. It is a story, told in part, through the device of a Journal as she might have written it being based on accumulated material unearthed from records, letters, and memorabilia.

The unfolding of Millie's story has enriched my own life as, inevitably, I became aware of similarities and dissimilarities between my Grandmother's character and my own.

As I remember her, my Grandmother was a realist; no romanticism, fancy furbelows or falsehood about her. She had the ability to recognize her own shortcomings. She could laugh at herself and she could cry. Her love of life became manifest in her appreciation of nature, her insatiable curiosity, her thirst for knowledge, her enjoyment of art and music.

Her faith in the art and science of healing was unshakable. Her comprehension of harmony grew as she confronted adversity and acted to overcome its evil.

Finally, her grandmotherly understanding evolved under the influence of daily contact with her five lively grandchildren.

PREAMBLE

A Joyless Christmas Morning in 1927

A telegram was delivered at our front door early on Christmas morning, 1927, sent by my Father who had the previous week left Syracuse with his parents to help them settle into their old North Carolina bungalow for the winter. Any telegram received by our family inevitably had a foreboding effect on the recipients — bad news. Slowly I read the words aloud to the stunned family as we were in the midst of opening presents.

CLASS OF SERVICE	WESTERN UNION	SYMBOLS
This is a full-rate Telegram or -Cablegram unless its deferred character is indicated by a suitable symbol above or preceding the address.		DL = Day Letter NL = Night Letter LC = Deferred Cable NLT = Cable Night Letter Ship Radiogram

The filing time shown in the date line on telegrams and day letters is STANDARD TIME at point of origin. Time of receipt is STANDARD TIME at point of destination

SUNDAY, DEC. 25, 1927

"GRANDMOTHER DEMOTT DIED PEACEFULLY THIS CHRISTMAS MORNING — STOP — WILL ARRIVE ON THE LATE TRAIN TUESDAY AFTERNOON WITH ANDREW — STOP — MOTHER'S BODY WILL BE TRANSPORTED DIRECTLY TO THE UNDERTAKER — STOP — DAD"

Suddenly there was a lasting pall over our Christmas Day.
After five o'clock Tuesday afternoon we all gathered in the darkened living room of our grandparents' red brick house await-

1

ing Dad's and Andrew's sad homecoming. The Grandfather's clock in its corner on the stair landing, was mute.

We sat silently for some time in the shadowed room, each immersed in peculiarly private thoughts. A newly laid fire in the hearth sputtered, sending sparks and smoke up the chimney. We had decided that Grandfather's arrival into our own Christmas bedecked house would be inappropriate. He would be more comfortable in his own home — cold as it was. A furnace fire had recently been coal-fed and prodded so that the radiators were just then beginning to cough, creak and whistle as the hot water began to circulate in them.

Aunt L. brought us face to face with present reality as she announced, "Well, I suppose I could get Amelia's burial clothes ready for the undertaker." Instantaneous vision of white Oriental embroidered silk flashed into my consciousness. I was thinking of the beautiful material my Grandmother had carried back from Japan many years ago with the promise she had given me that it would be saved for my wedding gown — but instead had been fashioned into a dress for her. It would be her shroud — not my wedding dress.

And then Auntie J. in her most lugubrious tone of voice, chanted "Well we all knew this was going to happen. I suppose we have known the worst for months. I just wonder how long Andrew can hold out without Millie . . . considering his urinary problems and all." Her knitting needles clicked on and on rhythmically.

A whining neighbor then voiced her concern about the funeral service, about food that should be provided, as she shook her head slowly from side to side.

We all sat quietly in the damp, chilly room. There seemed to be a noticeable lack of audible grief.

Young Frances, seated next to me on the floor, concentrating her gaze on the friendly old tiger skin spread out as if about to fall asleep by the hearth, muttered, "You know I have always hated our Grandmother." there was a hushed gasp.

"Why?" I asked her.

"Well," she continued, slowly choosing her words, "I'll never forget what she said about me when I was a little girl."

"What did she say?" I asked as I put my arm around her.

"I'll never forget it. Honney, once she said I had pig's eyes."

"What did she ever mean? You don't have pig's eyes!" I stared at her sharply. "Your eyes are your very own — like Andra's and mine — brown, like our Father's."

"Oh, it was the way she said it! . . . As if pig's eyes are small, mean. As if I had grown big and fat and homely and stupid like a pig . . . as if I reminded her of a pig the way I walk . . . as if she didn't like me at all. . . . Hardly anybody likes a pig! I don't think she ever liked me!"

I laughed. "Frances, it's funny but I can remember too when she said that. So long ago. You are wrong about what she meant. You didn't hear what else she said. She kept on talking about you after you and Andra had left the house."

"What else did she say? That I eat like a pig? Because I'm always hungry. That I'm sloppy as a pig? That I smell like a pig?"

"Oh no, Franny, stop it! You know how she used to talk — as if everyone should stop whatever they were doing and pay attention to her. What she really said was that the homeliest young children grow into the most beautiful young women and that she thought from her experience of observing families, that *you* would turn into the loveliest looking grown-up of all of us! And probably the nicest because you love flowers and birds — just as she always has!"

"Did she say that? Really?"

And then I remember after another sustained silence, Andra broke in as if she had just remembered something important.

"Hey, Everybody! I'm supposed to go to the movies with Bill on Thursday night. Do you suppose I could? I know the funeral is on that day. Should a funeral stop me from going to the movies if I want to go? . . . Well, I simply won't let it stop me! I really won't!

I don't care what Dad says."

And I remember the sound of two young lads' voices becoming increasingly shrill, strident, argumentative, finally exploding from the direction of the hall. Sounds of brotherly biffs until a small boy cried.

Silence again as the headlights of the taxi, veering into the driveway alerted us. Dad and Grandfather were home.

As I lighted the lamps, I was wondering what effect Grandmother's death would have on all our lives. My Grandfather's business. Would he stay north without Grandmother?

Where would he live? What would happen to the big red brick house? It would seem so very empty without her. I would never want a family of strangers living there. I thought about my Father's usual equinimity . . . and the lump in my own throat with a surge of outrage that my Grandmother would never respond to the Christmas letter I had written to her.

All thoughts were interrupted by the sudden appearance of faithful old Edith. She hobbled across the room balancing a huge tray heavy with a pitcher of hot mulled cider, cut glass punch cups, linen napkins and a large plate of sandwiches, another of her warm ginger cookies with raisins in the center. Carefully she set them on the oak library table as she looked sadly from one to the other of the family and neighbors—adults and children. She could not speak. Her eyes were swollen, blotched red, her face streaked with tears. She was weeping. Deep, gutteral sobs. The only sounds of grief in that cold, clammy room.

PART I

Millie's Birth, Education, Marriage and
Life as Mother and Teacher

PART I

The Grandfather clock standing in the corner of the parlor had already struck four times on the chilly morning of April 14, 1846 when my Grandmother, Amelia Eunice Lamb, was born in the village of Pompey Hill, New York—the second child and only daughter of Randolph Dyer Lamb, a farmer, and his wife Mary Randall Lamb. Forebears of both parents had been early settlers of the Massachusetts Bay Colony, having sailed from England in the mid-sixteeen hundreds. Children and grandchildren of those early settlers after the Revolutionary War were adventurous — adventurous and as brave as their forebears—as they trekked westward through Indian country, up hills, through valleys, cutting their way through great forests, fording streams on foot, on horseback, in oxen-drawn carts seeking new lands to settle.

The presence of mountains, rivers, lakes and swift-running streams lured those intrepid folk into areas of primeval wilderness. Together as family groups they cleared acres of land, using the trees they cut down as timber for building their log cabins and as fuel for heat and cooking. They dragged boulders from the fertile fields, utilizing the stones for walls and fences.

They plowed their fields, planted seeds and eventually acquired pigs, sheep, cattle, chickens and ducks. Through cooperative effort they raised up meeting houses similar to those they had left behind in New England. They built schools and places of worship. Towns multiplied as over the years the fertile fields expanded for many miles over the hilly central New York State countryside.

In 1776 the Continental Congress had proposed the establishment of land grants instead of money to be awarded surviving soldiers who had fought in the Revolutionary War. These lands were designated as "Gratuity Lands" to be awarded through the states by the federal government. Colonel John Lamb of Pompey who had commanded a regiment of artillery could have been assigned an allotment of 100 acres. However, I have found no record as to whether or not he ever actually received such land.

In March of 1781 and again in 1782 the New York State Legislature passed acts to induce more men to serve in defense of the country. An enlisted man was promised 500 acres of "Bounty Land" if he would serve three years. Officers would receive more according to their military rank. Land purchased in 1778 from the Onondaga Indians, known as the "Military Tract," was laid out in central New York State, originally containing 1,800,000 acres, exclusive of the Indian Reservations.

In 1794, at the same time that the county was designated as "Onondaga County," the town of Manlius came into existence being equal to 60,000 acres of the Military Tract. One of those lots, known on the official map as Manlius - Lot Number 68 - was drawn by Col. John Lamb. Among the family records this document has been preserved, but whether John Lamb used the land himself, exchanged it, sold it or passed it on to heirs or others is not known. Col. John Lamb did serve for six years as Supervisor of the Town of Pompey, beginning in 1797, and we know that Randolph and Mary Lamb years later lived with their family of two children in Pompey Hill. Zachary Taylor was president while another war was being fought between the United States and Mexico resulting finally in establishment of a recognized border — the Rio Grande — between the two countries. And there were only twenty-nine stars in the red, white and blue American flag: only twenty-nine states in our growing country.

When Amelia was five years old her father moved his family from the high hilly region of Pompey to the established township of Manlius where he now owned a larger farm that abutted a spring-fed swan pond. Many of the stories my Grandmother told

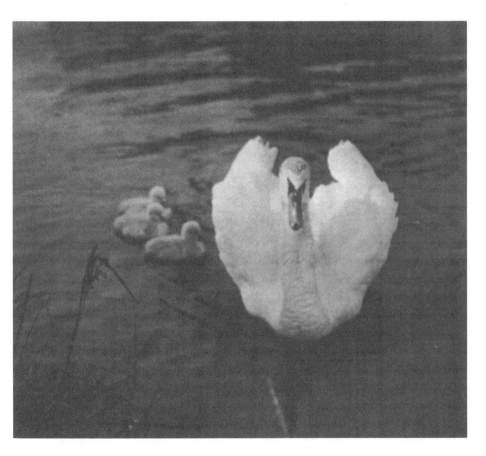

me reflected her life on that farm: her feeding of the swans, her catching fish, her skating on the frozen surface during the winter time. Once she fell into the cold water causing the interruption of her menstrual period — a memorable moment for her.

On that farm she had learned to ride a horse bareback and to milk a cow. As a young child she learned from her mother the names and songs of the birds, to recognize the wild flowers and trees. By the time she was eight years old she was responsible for feeding the chickens and helping care for the young farm stock.

Amelia and her older brother, Henry, as youngsters were pupils
in the one-room district "common school." It must have been at
about the age of seven or eight that she wrote her first composi-
tion, one that I recently found pasted into her old scrapbook.

SUMMER

SUMMER IS A VERY PLEASANT TIME OF THE
YEAR. BURDS SING. AND THE SQUIRRELS PLAY.
ALL NATUR LOOKS GAY. I LUV TO GO TO
SCHOOL. I LUV TO GO INTO THE WOODS TO
GATHER FLOWERS.
THE SQUIRRELS HOP LIKE GRAS HOPPERS. SOME
BOYS KILL THE BURDS AND THE SQUIRRELS.
I THINK THE GOLDFINCH IS THE PRETTYEST
BURD. THIS IS BECAUSE HE IS YELLOW ALL
OVER.

Later on Henry and Amelia studied at the Manlius Academy
where their parents paid a small tuition fee. When Amelia, or
Millie, as she was called by her friends, was sixteen, Henry, nineteen, enlisted in the Union Army as a musician. He was assigned
as a cornetist with the New York Cavalry Band a year after the
bombardment of Fort Sumter at Charleston, South Carolina in
1861. Amelia saved the many letters her brother had written to
her during the war describing his various assignments and adventures within the country both north and south of the Mason Dixon
Line.

Among these letters was one written at the time of the assassi-
nation of President Lincoln, April 14, 1865, Amelia's nineteenth
birthday. It was mailed from General Washburn's Headquarters
at Memphis, Tennessee. This was his letter:

Dear Sister,

Here it has been nothing but mourning and the sound of
dirges ever since the news came of President LINCOLN'S

death. Was that not an awful thing? This city of Memphis is
hung in mourning. I suppose it is so throughout the United
States. Last Monday all the troops in this district—citizens and
all turned out to meet in mourning. They formed one grand
procession headed by the Post Band. We were all mounted on
white mares. The bridles were trimmed with crepe—white and
black. I am sending the program of all activities to Pa.

Black crepe was hung on all our instruments and around our
left arms. I tell you we looked nice. There is no other band
capable of performing in parade as we can. We play some
splendid dirges and we handle them well. Guns were fired here
all day from the Batteries and the Fort every half hour and
church bells were tolled. All places of business were closed and
everything looked mournful.

Do you think they will ever find the assassins? I hope they do.
Hon. Andrew Johnson from Tennessee is now the President. I
hope he will prove to be a good man, especially at this time.

Lincoln's death causes great excitement here among the
soldiers. It is hard to keep them from shooting anyone unless he
is known to be loyal.

There were four citizens shot here by our soldiers last Sunday
for expressing sentiments of disloyalty. The official order now is
to take no prisoners.

Every man who is found taking up arms against the Union
government is to be shot or hung. Sometimes our men suffer as
much as the Rebs.

Six men of our Regiment were murdered in cold blood yesterday after they were taken prisoners by General Forrest's
men. While our men were on patrol near Germantown about
50 miles from here, Forrest's soldiers pitched into them.
Immediately about 5000 of our Cavalry dashed after General
Forrest, the Reb leader.

Tomorrow we are ordered again with the Military and the
Masons of this city to play again. We are to be mounted at
General Washburn's headquarters early in the morning.

Tell Pa I am sending him a Memphis news paper. We are all
well. Write often.

Henry D. Lamb

P.S. Today is a pleasant day to go swiming skinny-wise.

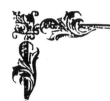

Funeral Hymn.

TO BE SUNG BY THE PHILHARMONIC SOCIETY.

Mourn for the living, mourn ;
    But weep not for the dead ;
They need your tears from whom is torn
    Their patern and their head.

But he, the suffering saint,
    To whom release is given,
No tongue can tell, no fancy paint,
    His joy and peace in heaven.

Mourn for the living, mourn,
    For they have lost a friend,
Whose spirit is by angels borne
    Where Unions have no end.

Pray for the living, pray ;
    Besiege the throne of God :
That all may seek the upward way
    His careful footsteps trod.

Let faith and hope to birth
    In every heart arise,
That those who mourn his loss on earth,
    May join him in the skies.

AMERICA.

[Gen. Washburn desires all to join in singing
this beautiful anthem.]

My country ! 'tis of thee,
Sweet land of liberty !
    Of thee I sing ;
        Land where my fathers died ;
        Land of the pilgrim's pride ;
        From every mountain side,
    Let freedom ring.

My native country ! thee,
Land of the noble free,
    Thy name I love ;
        I love thy rocks and rills,
        Thy woods and templed hills ;
        My heart with rapture thrills,
    Like that above.

Our father's God ! to thee,
Author of liberty !
    To thee we sing ;
        Long may our land be bright,
        With freedom's holy light,
        Protect us by thy might,
    Great God, our King !

It was not until after the end of the war that Henry was mustered out of the service. He returned to the family farm at Manlius, but was depressed and discontented with farm life. Many of his friends had either been killed, wounded or had moved west to find employment. Henry too headed for the big city of Chicago with the hope that his unpleasant memories would fade as he explored new horizons.

After graduation from the Academies in Manlius and then in nearby Fayetteville as well, Millie left home for further study and teacher training in Oswego, New York. Courses there included advanced work in mathematics and science as well as more Latin and further reading of Greek mythology and world history, as well as in penmanship and art. With these studies completed, she would be well prepared to take a position as a teacher.

By the time she was twenty-one years old she returned to Manlius to be assistant principal and teacher in the Union school, located near the farm in the country district. That summer at a church picnic she met a young man who had come from Hillsboro, New York, north of Oneida Lake, to master the art of woodworking at a local Manlius wagon shop. He was Edward Dann, the youngest son of a large family whose older brothers had all moved from the big farm to settle as carriage builders in Connecticut.

In accordance with the ways of youth, Edward and Millie became profoundly attracted to each other and determined by the end of the year to marry the following March. This was during a time when the entire country was enmeshed in financial, industrial and political upheaval. The former slaves, now freed, were being gradually assimilated into a new way of life both north and south of the Mason Dixon Line.

For many years Millie kept a poem Edward had composed for her during the time of their courtship. In reading it, there can be no doubt of his devotion to her, yet the poem seems strangely ironic.

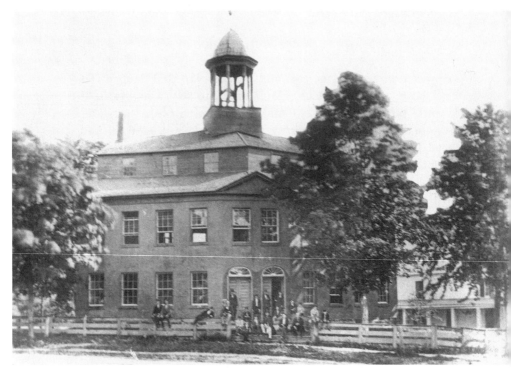

Manlius Academy with Millie as a student, 1861-1863.

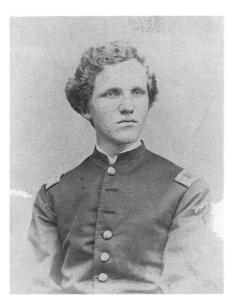

Millie's brother Henry in Civil War uniform, 1865.

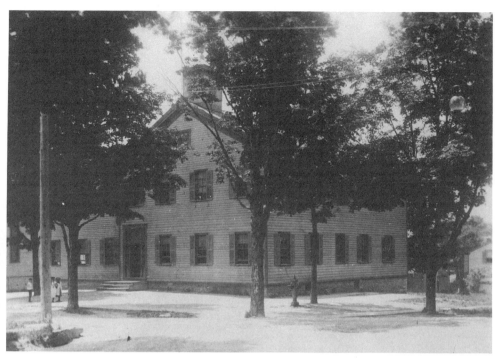

Manlius Union School where Millie taught and was assistant to the Principal, 1866-1868. (This and Manlius Academy photograph courtesy of Manlius Historical Society.)

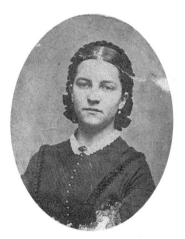

Millie as a teacher.

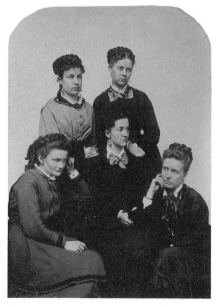

Millie with four of her unidentified friends.

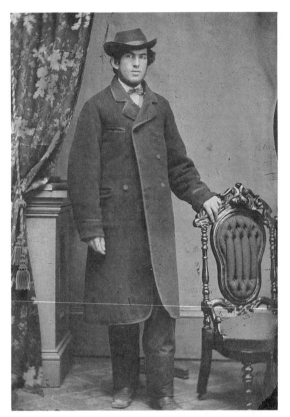

Edward Howard Dann, the bridegroom, 1868.

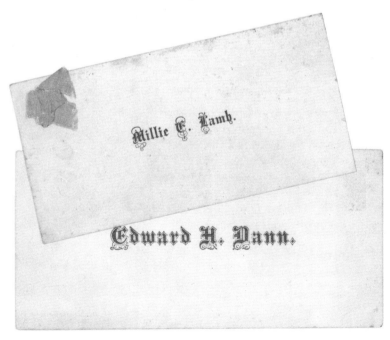

Cards announcing the engagement of Edward and Millie.

TO MILLIE

I wish thee Gentle Girl, a life
From sorrows blight, as free
As here midst darkness, tears of strife
Earth's pilgrimage may be.
Let no dark cloud of trouble rise
With frowning brow severe
To shroud in gloom thy sunny skies
To cause a flowing tear.

But let those eyes through lengthened years
Their living light retain
Unknown to grief, undimm'd by tears —
Sore tears for others' pain.
And long may time consent to spare
The sweetly blooming rose
That on thy cheek — untouched by care —
Its tempting beauty glows.

I wish for thee — the boon is rare —
The choicest Heaven bestows —
A Friend to share thy every care
To soften all thy woes.
A Friend whom thou shalt ever find
In sunshine and in gloom
Devoted, constant, ever kind
As during love's young bloom.

And more dear Girl, I wish thee more
Than this poor world can give:
I wish for thee when life is o'er
A home where angels live.
A home where wearied spirits rest.
Where hearts forget to ache,
Where all are freely, freely blest.
Where friends no more foresake.

And further on in the same notebook, these words appeared still clear in her own Spencerian script:

> "Can you conceive of anything better, finer, dearer than the home of married love? Its brief partings almost sweet because they point to an early reunion—its new and bewildering emotions, its common interests, its hours so dream-like—yet so real, the sympathy of mirth, the sympathy of grief, the delicious mystery of affection binding heart to heart, the perfect non-reserve yet the perfect reverence for each other. . . . This realization must be ours."

Amelia Eunice Lamb and Edward Howard Dann were married March 24, 1868 at two o'clock in the afternoon in the little white Presbyterian church in Manlius with the Reverend Herbert Graley officiating. He had been minister and friend of the Lamb family since their early days of living in Pompey Hill.

I still have in my possession a small gold-embossed, leather book entitled "A Christian Minister's Affectionate Advice to a Married Couple." Included within its binding was a certificate of the marriage of Mr. Edward H. Dann and Miss Millie E. Lamb at Manlius, New York on March 24, 1868.

Pastor Alfred Graley addressed the couple in a friendly, personal fashion: "The marriage relationship is the most important of any you are capable of forming in this life. . . . It is a union constituted not merely for the reciprocal benefit of two persons who agree to form it, but likewise for the benefit of society. . . . You are fellow-travellers on the road of life. You have pledged yourselves to bear each other's burdens, to respect each other's peace of mind.

"Trials and difficulties are the common lot of humanity. Rough roads, dark nights and stormy days are to be expected. . . . Communication contributes to the warmth of mutual affection, to generous confidence one toward the other. Expect to discover faults in each other.

"Society takes its character from qualities brought into being through those qualities developed in the home. Respect your time together as a family in that home."

Reverend Graley reminded the wife that she had vowed to honor the will of her husband. He also forcefully urged the husband to seek his wife's opinions, and to consider her as a cherished, trustworthy partner.

He charged them both to regard the institution of marriage as a foundation for enhancing and developing their love for each other.

The families of both the bride and groom had joined to give their blessings and with friends and other relatives met together at the church to wish the couple future happiness.

Village officials, farmers and their wives, storekeepers and the owner of the wagon shop where Edward had been employed, were present at the marriage ceremony. There were little children, as well as the older pupils from Millie's country school, teachers and "soldier boys" safely home from the war — all bidding the bride and groom a clamorous farewell. After a last gathering up of their gifts and belongings at the farmhouse they bundled into a bright bow-bedecked horse-drawn sleigh, bells jingling. They were off to the depot at Manlius Station (now Minoa) where the train for Syracuse was just about to leave.

There, with all their baggage stashed away, they hustled into their seats on the crowded train. Honeymoon-bound, the New York Central engine, gradually gathering speed, steamed along beneath white puffs of smoke toward Albany.

The following day they boarded the Hudson River steamboat for the cold trip down the river to New York City. After spending two days sight-seeing, they were once again passengers — this time aboard the Long Island ferry boat headed toward New Haven,

Connecticut.

Edward's brothers and their wives, who had lived in New Haven for several years, met the couple at the harbor wharf, drove them in their carriage behind a span of two white horses to the house on Greene Street where they would take possession of the upper flat. Brother William had only recently renovated the house, choosing to occupy the first floor with his growing family.

Snow was falling that cold March day as they entered the house. My Grandmother remembered the aroma of Scotch broth — her favorite soup — that was simmering on the coal stove as they entered their new home. The four rooms, neatly furnished, were far more beautiful than they had expected and there in the bedroom was a four-poster carved oak bed freshly made up with a blue and white quilted coverlet. To Edward and Millie, their future seemed rainbow blessed.

Edward was scheduled to begin work the following week with his five older brothers at the downtown manufacturing plant, The Dann Brothers Carriage Company. Each day Edward used his new woodworking skills at the factory as Millie exposed herself to the mysteries of housekeeping and planned a spring flower garden to be planted at the rear of the house.

Together they met their neighbors and explored the city — an enlightening experience since neither of them had ever lived beyond the boundary of farm or village. They learned to sail in the protected harbor. They fished from the pier. They took long walks up the trail to the top of East Rock.

Very soon they agreed that New Haven was a perfect place to make their home and in which to raise a family — as residents of this famous University town with its elm tree-lined streets, its harbor, its many parks, its central Green shadowed by Yale College spires and rooftops, its churches, its schools, its guardian red cliffs of towering East and West Rock.

During that year of 1868, President Andrew Johnson was impeached, tried and finally acquitted for attempting to remove from office his Secretary of War, Edwin Stanton, a defender of

the rights of slaveholders and for courageously supporting reconstruction of the Southern States. Congressional impeachment
proceedings failed, Stanton resigned and returned to his law
practice. With a new Secretary of War, Johnson resumed his position as President. General Ulysses S. Grant was elected to the
presidency to succeed him in 1869 and remained in office for two
terms.

Serious challenges faced the people of the United States, with
problems ranging from domestic to public life nationwide. The
struggle identified in the newspapers as the Period of Reconstruction, required the strength, intelligence and imagination of everyone — the rich and the poor alike.

Edward and Millie became, as co-founders of another pioneer
family, adverturers into a changing era.

In July a letter arrived from Edward's sister, Esther, poignantly
describing life back at the Dann family farm:

Camden, N.Y.
July 3, '68

Dear Brother and Sister,

Millie, I think that if you were to visit me now you would
enjoy it better than when you were here last winter. It is indeed
very pleasant here during the summer season. And my dear
Brother it affords us a great deal of pleasure to hear that you
are so happy in your own home. Do you go into town very
often?

It is after ten o'clock. All except me have retired. It is such a
beautiful moonlit eve I enjoy being up.

Father is going to write to our brother John in the morning. I
was delighted with the plan that brothers John, Jesse and
William proposed about buying this farm, but so far Father
does not say much. Says there will have to be a change in the
fall. I so often think of the good times we used to have when
Edward was at home. When I see my friends with good kind

brothers at home I almost envy them.

Have you had any pictures taken since you went to New Haven? If so I shall have to remind you of your promise to send us one.

Mr. Wood has asked me to teach school in the town but I could not be spared from home. He said they would pay any wages I would ask.

How do you like keeping house, Millie? Do you get along nicely with the baking? And do you get lonesome for your old Manlius home? Please write to us. Just take time and write! I must stop. We shall miss you on the Fourth—tomorrow when I shall make the strawberry shortcake. I wish you were both here to have dinner with us. Today has been the most sultry day I most ever saw. I took my lunch into the woods and read all afternoon.

I will close now wishing for you both all the happiness possible in the connubial state.

Ever, your affectionate Sister

Esther

As the summer had enticed them to take short exploratory trips into the countryside of Connecticut, so did autumn and winter draw Edward and Millie into excursions with family and friends. Thanksgiving and Christmas involved them in unfamiliar New England customs and the warmth of genuine family conviviality.

They were acutely aware of the new chapter in their marriage which was about to become reality. Early in the new year a child would be born to them—a new beginning.

To celebrate their first Christmas together they had planned one mutual present to celebrate Millie's pregnancy. Edward had handcrafted a cradle from hard maple wood, had rubbed it with wax until it shone. Beautiful and strong it was, with rockers. Millie, discovering talent she never knew she possessed, had fashioned a sturdy mattress and cover so that with the baby presents they had received, this first child of theirs was already assured a warm welcome.

Millie had confided in her favorite sister-in-law that she was becoming more and more eager to see, to hold, to love, to care for their first-born child.

It was not enough to feel the strengthening movements within her, the tiny punches, the stretching, even the unborn baby's hiccoughs. Dr. Lyons, who had been caring for her, promised that he would be around at the time of her labor. Anne and Sarah, as caring sisters-in-law, had assured her they would be there by her side for comfort also.

In January Millie and Edward had attended several parties in spite of the fact that Millie knew there were raised eyebrows among their friends who were skeptical of her appearance in public so late in her pregnancy.

She wrote to her Mother that even Edward assumed a father-to-be look of pride. Millie spoke freely of the increased vigor she felt: perceptions more acute, colors brighter, the cold more energizing.

Then suddenly their life changed—unexpectedly. In mid-January, Edward, the physically strong, lithe, intensely caring young husband lay burning with fever beside Millie. He wanted no food. Only water—more water. During the day he thrashed about the bed as if he were having a nightmare. Millie had never seen an illness like this. She tried to comfort him. Her efforts were useless. As night darkened the room it seemed to her that he was breathing with difficulty, that physically he was weaker.

She became worried, called William's wife from downstairs, confided her fears. William would get the doctor. But Dr. Lyons was tending a sick child and would be unable to make the house call until tomorrow. Millie sat beside her husband with tears in her eyes. She had never felt so powerless—so frustrated by ignorance.

As dawn began to light New Haven, the bare branches of the elm tree at the side of the house cast a menacing lacy black shadow through the window onto the bed. Edward drowsed.

Early in the morning Doctor Lyons arrived. Millie thought as she greeted him that he had probably had no sleep himself. He was carrying his black bag which seemed to Millie to be mysteriously endowed with medical magic. The doctor pressed and probed Edward's tender turgid abdomen as he sought to elicit answers from him. Only a groan from Edward—a shudder. Writhing in agony, he managed to turn his entire body toward the wall . . . and vomited blood. As Millie stood by the bed watching his painful ordeal, the child within her seemed at the very moment to be brusquely changing position. Millie felt a sharp pain. She gasped as she pressed her hands instinctively and protectively onto her abdomen.

At the door the doctor put his arm about Millie's shoulders and told her that Edward was suffering from typhoid fever. There was an epidemic in the city. She must stay with him, watch him day and night, keep cool compresses on his forehead, give him only liquids by mouth, keep a record of the frequency of vomiting and diarrhea, be alert if signs of dementia should occur, call for help if she became frightened. He also assured her that her baby was not yet ready to be born.

The need to give her love to Edward burgeoned to crescendo intensity—a passionate frustration.

On January twelfth a letter came from Edward's father who at the time did not know of his son's illness. He wrote of the hard times on the farm with only his wife and two daughters to help him with the barn chores. His three older sons had decided not to assume responsibility for the farm. He complained that "my lims are growing stiff and weak and that considering the situation, dear Edward, I would be glad to have you come back to take my place." He added "farming is a slow way to make money but it is a sure way to live by." He reminisced about the dryness of the summer which had resulted in a light harvest of hay, insufficient for the large herd of cattle he must feed this winter.

He thanked God that both he and Mary were now in good health. He was proud of his sons' successes at the factory but was concerned for his and Mary's future. He could not envision life

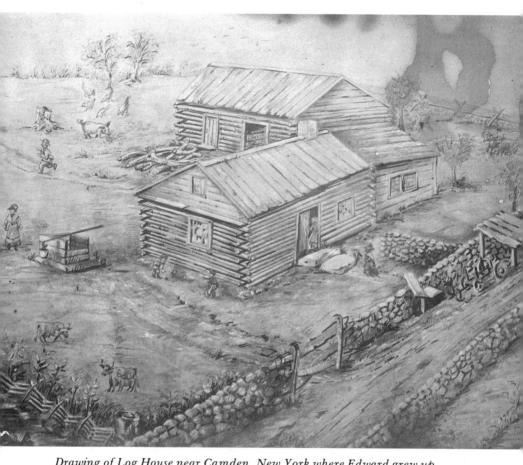

Drawing of Log House near Camden, New York where Edward grew up.
(Drawn by John Dann, Edward's father, circa 1860.)

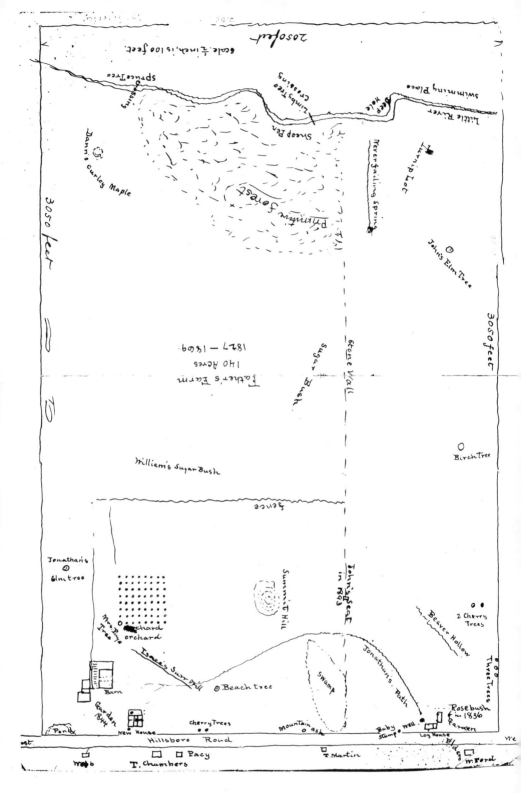

Drawing of the Dann farm (Drawn by John Dann, Edward's father, circa 1860.)

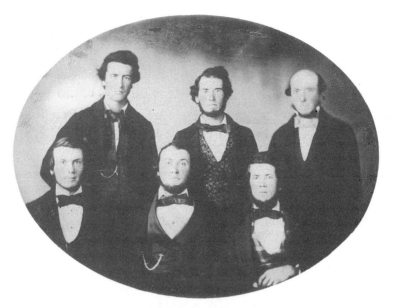

The six Dann brothers when Dann Brothers Manufacturing Company was established in New Haven, Connecticut, 1858.

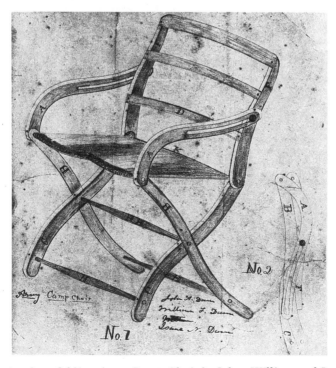

Design for a folding Army Camp Chair by John, William and Isaac. Theirs was the first folding chair and the Dann Brothers manufactured it for the army.

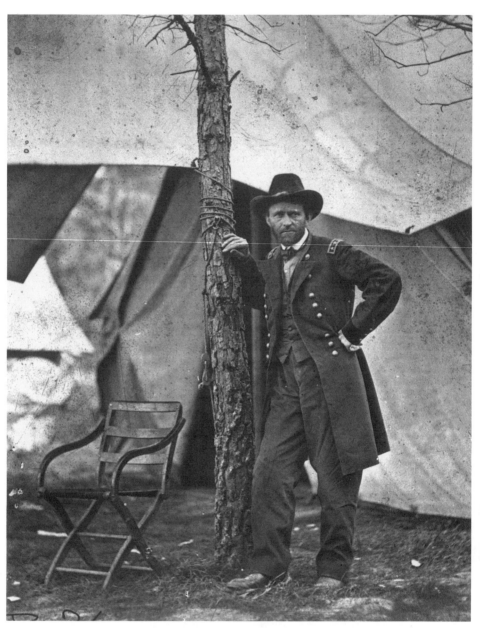

General Ulysses S. Grant with one of the chairs beside his tent.
(Courtesy of the National Achives, Washington, D.C.)

away from the farm he loved.

Millie read the letter to her husband although she knew he was incapable of completely comprehending the heart of the message. Edward had told her many personal stories about his family's farm. His father, who had migrated from Ireland early in the century, had landed in Montreal. Eventually he had found his way on foot along Lake Champlain to central New York State.

Following marriage to young Mary MacPherson, Edward's parents settled on the farm they had purchased near the town of Camden, north of Oneida Lake. There they raised their eleven sons and daughters to adulthood. One small boy of two years, who had been the twelfth child, died of whooping cough. He was buried in the nearby church yard.

Edward's mother, Mary, born in Scotland, was a weaver. She spun and wove cloth for clothing and bedding from cotton; for coats and blankets and rugs she spun and wove from the wool of the sheep they raised. Their land produced fruits and vegetables and grain both to sell and for their own use.

Edward had told Millie about his early adventures on the Little River running at the south edge of the property. It provided fish. There was swimming in summer and skating in winter. Meat on the farm was processed from the sheep, pigs and chickens they raised. Cattle provided milk, cream for butter, meat at slaughtering time. John Dann became adept at fashioning rough shoes for his family from the animal hides. Wood as fuel for heating and cooking had to be hewn and hauled from the forest behind the log cabin, weaving house and barn. Edward had grown up accustomed to hard work and loyalty to family

Within a few days after the arrival of his father's letter, Edward seemed to rally a bit.

He sweated profusely and wanted food. He was determined to return to his work at the carriage plant. Prior to his sickness he had been intent on repairing an old sleigh. It had been severely seared in a horse barn fire. He kept mumbling incoherently about the beauty of its bent wood frame, its runners, its unique design.

When Millie refused to give him his clothes he became obsessed with the need to find his tools. Crazed, no longer her lover, no longer her calm, stalwart Edward, he behaved like a mad man. They were each—husband and wife—mentally manacled by the awful curse of Edward's illness.

Gradually Edward became too weak to continue his fight for life. He was dying. There was a blurred aura about him—even his eyes that had so often lit up with love for her were veiled, unseeing. At moments before seven o'clock the morning of January 24th, Edward died. Millie had never before witnessed death except among the animals on her father's Manlius farm. She fought the numbness, the grief that engulfed her.

The obituary from the New Haven newspaper reported:

> There was an unusually large attendance at St. John's Methodist Church yesterday afternoon, the occasion being the funeral of EDWARD HOWARD DANN of this city.
>
> He was the youngest son of John and Mary Dann of Camden, N.Y., 27 years of age. He is survived besides his wife, by six brothers and four sisters. Just ten months previous to the day of his burial, he was married in the town of Manlius, New York to Miss Amelia Lamb who now mourns a good, affectionate and Christian husband.

This account and a copy of the funeral service she saved together with a snip of cedar which had rested with flowers on the casket.

After the funeral and hasty packing, Millie bade the new family she had so wholeheartedly adopted, a sad farewell. Accompanied by her brother Henry, who had come for the funeral, Millie returned by train to her parents' home in the hamlet of Kirkville, New York. The Manlius farm, where Millie and Henry had grown up, had only recently been sold after the retirement of their parents. Millie had never seen the new cottage where she hoped there would be room enough for her, the little Christmas cradle and her soon-to-be-born babe.

Millie had faced one challenge after another. Just two weeks after the funeral of her husband, on February 7, 1869, young Teddy was born in the bedroom of her parents' home—a healthy, well-formed, lustily-crying child.

Within a few months Millie began to look for means of helping to support herself and the baby. Having had training in painting and artcraft, she set about establishing herself as a home teacher for the ladies of the village and the countryside. She taught china painting, oil picture painting and the art of arranging dried flowers and stalks of grain to be framed behind glass. At the time another form of art had become popular. Ladies made use of wax to form flowers, leaves, wreaths, and religious symbols. A favorite model demonstrated the mounting of a solid wax cross on a firm wax base, the cross being draped with wax ivy as a symbol of everlasting life, to commemorate the death of a family member. The art form was then preserved under a glass bell jar or framed in a shadow box to be displayed in a Victorian parlor.

Millie noticed that in the local Manlius newspaper printed once a week that there was seldom any item of interest from neighboring Kirkville. Gathering her wits and courage she stopped at the news office one morning and asked to see the publisher. Recognizing the Lamb in her name, the editor* invited her to sit down at the other side of his desk piled high with news items. She asked him if he would be interested in hiring a reporter from the Kirkville area.

She explained that there were lectures often delivered at the Union Church in Kirkville which might be of general interest. She spoke about local comings and goings since the town was located centrally—important both as a canal boat stop and a depot for the New York Central Railroad.

She proposed a column—one which she would assume responsibility for writing and submitting on time. The editor explained

* F. A. Darling, a newcomer as a business man, arrived in 1866 to take over the publishing of the weekly paper.

that most of the work for the paper was being done by men but if she were willing to use a pseudonym such as "Country Cousin" he would be willing to give her a try. This was another job she could accomplish at home. And so it was that the "Country Cousin from Kirkville" came into being.

For several years the *Recorder* printed Millie's column of folksy news — descriptions of gala gatherings, rural calamities, births, deaths, illnesses, real estate transactions, store openings and closings, the need for new sidewalks, politics and women's rights — all with the byline of Country Cousin.

Typical of the column she wrote came from the following accounts found in her own scrapbook:

To the Editor of the Weekly Recorder — From Kirkville 1871

First week in April — moving week in the country. Mud-mud-mud - cross women - crying babies - cold dinners. C.B. Johnson has sold his farm of forty acres to George Dominick for $4,000. Mr. George Cook who has long been a resident of Kirkville has left us to find a home in Fayetteville.

Lawrence Bartlett intends to leave us to attend school at Oneida Seminary, preparatory to teaching. Miss Sarah Hay of Fayetteville will teach our district school the coming season. We wish her success.

Our cheese factory will recommence operation on the 11th. It is to be hoped that the good reputation the factory has acquired will be maintained.

Mr. James Snow who has been sick for several weeks, still lies in critical condition.

Mr. Patrick, our obliging depot agent, lost a valuable horse last week, thus breaking up his fine span. Mr. John Van-Antwerp has rented and reopened the Canal Grocery. Mr. Hoag has just received a fine stock of boots and shoes for all members of the family. Daily he expects more. Give Charley a call — he never fails to give feet a good fit at a reasonable price.

The rain continues — drizzle, drizzle, drizzle — mud and more mud. The cold wet weather has hindered many farmers from sowing their grain and getting to their other spring work. But we all know that we have been promised a "seed time" and we believe that proper time will come.

Country Cousin

And another example:

August 22, 1871

To the Editor of the Weekly Recorder:

Within the past two weeks, scarlet fever has raged here fearfully. The Norman Clocks have lost a daughter and another child, a son, was so near death as to be totally blind. We have learned today that his condition is much improved.

The numerous friends of Miss Libbie Adams will be pleased to learn that she is slowly recovering from the same dreadful fever. No new cases have so far been reported.

Last evening Mrs. Matilda Gage, proponent of women's suffrage and a resident of Fayetteville, addressed the people of this place at the Union Church on the subject of Votes for Women. There was a good attendance and we think that those who attended came away with different ideas and less prejudice on the subject than they came with. Mrs. Gage spoke well and handled the question with force and ability. Concerning our sidewalks which are in such deplorable condition, she assured us that it is the ballot which can implement the building of sidewalks. We needn't wonder what causes them NOT to be built. We want to assure Mrs. Gage that if the women of Kirkville had the use of the ballot as the men in our village do, our sidewalks would no longer disgrace us.

The shin-scratching, neck-breaking, nose-smashing, decayed old planks would be ripped up and replaced with a decent sidewalk. We believe that surely the day will come that the ballot will be entrusted to woman and that she will be educated to use it properly.

Your Country Cousin

In 1872 with powerful encouragement from both her parents,

Millie decided to apply for a teaching position in the Syracuse public school system. It involved a move to the city for her, allowing time to spend with Teddy and her parents only on weekends and vacations. The child at three-and-a-half was an active, imaginative youngster — a drain on the strength of his grandparents. Their discipline was strict, their hearts loving. Millie's being able to take full responsibility and care of the boy during the summer months made the over-all plan feasible.

And so it was that in September Millie began teaching third grade in Putnam School, not far from where she was boarding in the city of Syracuse.

From her scrapbook comes this poem, author unknown:

THE SCHOOL TEACHER

Fifty little urchins
Coming through the door
Pushing, crowding, making
A terrific roar.

Fifty little pilgrims
On their way to fame:
If they fail to make it,
Who will be to blame?

High and lowly stations,
Birds of every feather
On a common level
Here are brought together.

Dirty little faces, loving little hearts,
Eyes brimful of mischief, well skilled in all the arts,
Boots and shoes a-shuffling, slates and books a-rattling.
In the corner yonder two pugilists a-battling.
Parents say their children should mind their p's and q's,
In school their brilliant talents should never be abused.

Ah - To be a teacher!

At the end of three years of teaching in the Syracuse Public School System, Millie became seriously ill. She appealed to one of the leading physicians of the city who explained to her that she must not return to Kirkville. Dr. VanDuyn confirmed her worst fear—that she was suffering from typhoid fever, the deadly disease which had developed epidemic proportion. Immediately he made preparation for her to be admitted to the hospital, formerly called the "City Pest House" where he would continue caring for her.

A stolid white-uniformed woman wheeled her down a long dark corridor lined with typhoid victims. Sounds of retching, coughing, moaning. Cots on either side of the ward were occupied by women—all in varying stages of the disease. The stench of death pervaded. At one empty cot, its covers neatly folded at the foot, the nurse stopped, helped Millie out of the wheelchair, directed her to disrobe and put on the clean muslin half-gown lying on the pillow. "Wait," she said. "The doctor will see you when he can. I don't know when that will be. There, now lie quietly and try to be patient. There is water on your little side table." With a drawn, weary smile she turned away, pushing the empty wheelchair to the entrance where the next victim was already awaiting admission.

Millie, shaking with fever and fear, curled herself into a tight miserable nonentity. Her hot tears blotted her pillow. Time became for her an eternity as the days and nights blurred into the coursing of a month. During moments of regaining full consciousness she vowed to herself that she would keep breathing, that she would not die. The vow intensified as she began to improve. She realized that she was twenty-nine years old, about the same age as Edward when typhoid fever claimed him as its victim. The awful memory. Teddy and her parents needed her. She must live! The pain, the chills and high fever, the difficulty in swallowing, the witnessing of death—these sensations broke into moments of mental clarity like distorted dreams. They would not fade as they wove themselves into the fabric of her memory. She tried to leave her cot, to escape her prison. Her legs seemed weighted down as if by lead. A nightmare. Her head ached, her eyes would not focus. She shuddered. Was this punishment by medieval torture? Had she been transported backward into the Dark Ages of history to be held prisoner for the rest of her life? She wanted to scream, but the sound that came from her throat was an unearthly moan. Tears and the acrid smell of her own sweat bathed her body. Improvement came slowly.

When the time came finally for her discharge, Dr. VanDuyn sat beside her cot. He talked with her about the successful battle she had fought. There were days when he admitted that even he doubted that she would recover.

She asked questions of him, no longer rambling in an unintelligible babble. She wanted to know more about the history of the old Pest House and this new facility, who the doctors were who were responsible for its administration and supervision. What role did the city fathers assume; was it run by a Board of Health as the schools were under the Board of Education? Her eyes caught his directly. She spoke with a fervor he had never before detected. In response, the tone of his voice changed. As she held out her hand to take his in a gesture of gratitude for his faithful overseeing of her care, he smiled not as a doctor to his patient, but as friend to friend and said, "Millie, *you should become a physician.*"

On a Red Letter Day of July as Millie continued to recuperate she did apply and was accepted as a member of the class to enter Syracuse University Medical School in September 1875, the college having been officially established for only three years at the time.

PART II

Millie's Journal Accounts of Medical School
in the 1870's and Her Practice Specializing
in the Care of Women Patients

PART II

Fifty years after Millie had been discharged from her long siege of battling to survive typhoid fever in 1875, her memories of the hospital for Infections Diseases (formerly known as the Pest House) were still vivid. And so were the five decades of her life which had intervened.

It was on a warm September afternoon in 1926 that my Grandmother and I picked ripe apples in the orchard behind the red brick house. Low branches heavy with fruit arched over the ground. The good smell of apples permeated the air as the two-handled wicker basket filled to overflowing.

With the basket swung low between us, we two—Grandmother and Granddaughter—walked slowly to the kitchen. Once there my Grandmother, obviously short of breath, slumped into the black Boston rocking chair next to the window. Soon, recovering her composure and with a sparkle in her eyes, she announced that she wanted to check something in the attic. Together we climbed the two flights of back stairs, stopping often.

The attic was a familiar place to me as I recalled using it as a secret hide-away for games of hide-and-seek only a few years ago. Old furniture was stored there, cobwebs hung in profusion, flies buzzed. There was a smell of musty paper and old wood. Rolls of unused wallpaper were coiled under the eaves, next to stacks of old magazines—*Ladies Home Journals* and *Saturday Evening Posts*. The old dress-up trunk was still there. The place was steamy hot.

Half limping to a far corner, near a window, my Grandmother

located a group of wooden crates and cardboard boxes heavily camouflaged with dust. As she pulled them out, bright sunbeams shafted through the disturbed particles of dust. Seated on an old three-legged stool, she pried the first box open. A new smell—old leather rotting. Beads of sweat stood out on her forehead and arms.

She was smiling as she opened old record books, notebooks filled with finely scribed notes and illustrations. One by one she opened boxes of letters, old obstetrical instruments, photograph albums, scrapbooks. In one large box lay her brother Henry's Civil War uniform, complete with blue-visored cap and sheathed saber.

A nostalgic tone slowed her speech as she spoke about a concern she had recently felt toward these remnants of another life. "They are my memories," she explained. "Who else would want to shuffle through them? I have been wondering what if there were a fire in this house or just suppose Grandfather and I die. All this mess would be so much more for someone to dispose of."

"Honney, I am going to ask you to take them to your house. Keep them. Perhaps someday you may find what is written of interest to you. . . . Perhaps."

So it was that I became the unconcerned keeper of my grandmother Millie's memorabilia for more than fifty years.

Millie's story today reflects the bringing to light of these memorabilia described in view of the times during which she lived.

THE JOURNAL BEGINS

I have determined today September 1, 1875 to begin a non-coercive Journal while I am in Medical School. Perhaps I'll keep it up afterwards as well. There are bound to be incidents, crises, frustrations, happenings which I should record. Right now I don't have a "best friend" to share a confidence with, one whom I could unburden a confidence.

It occurs to me that I might invent that best friend in the guise of my Journal to go through Medical School with me, to bear with me. Even when time is almost nonexistent my friend-to-be can be at hand.

As Teddy grows older, I can keep track of his development, his interests, his accomplishments. I'll forget details if I don't plan to keep a skeleton of a record.

It will also give me an outlet for expressing some of the thoughts I don't want to talk about. Right now I sense a tantalizing guilt. There are conflicts developing in my life that I must eventually face. What effect will this decision of mine to study day after day have on my boy? Will what I am doing bring my parents to an early death? Am I being sufficiently considerate of them in expecting them to move from farm to city at this time in their lives, to continue being "grandparents-in-charge?"

Do I, in truth, have faith in my professed religion? Discordant within me are unadmitted antagonisms, animosities, doubts. How strong must I prove myself to be? Am I intellectually equal to the mastery of medicine, to scholastic competition?

Sometimes I wonder now if I have forgotten how to sing, to dance, to laugh.

Already I have begun my Journal!

September 2, 1875

Now that I have had a rare second cup of coffee for breakfast I feel like gathering my thoughts as I sit looking out on the broad field behind my parents' little house in Kirkville. The trees are beginning to take on their fall brilliance, there is a smell of new-mown hay, asters are in bloom in the garden—the purples, the whites, the pinks. And I am keenly aware that the next installment of my life is looming.

Saying goodbye to my class of children, the other teachers and my friends at school last June left me both jubilant and sorrowful. At that time I didn't realize that I would not be returning to Putnam School as a teacher.

During the summer came my battle with typhoid fever in that hell hole of a Pest House. Scars will remain with me for my lifetime.

Physically I am thin, drained of strength and almost bald. The surprise is that my hair is now growing back curly!

The month of recuperation here in Kirkville with Teddy and my parents has been a blessing. After Brother Henry had left for the West and I had married and gone to New Haven to live several years ago, Mother and Pa decided it was time for them to retire from farming in Manlius. To cut down on their many responsibilities they determined to concentrate their most precious belongings into this tiny cottage here in neighboring Kirkville. And then—What irony! I arrived back home and young Teddy was born right here in this crowded cottage after my brief eleven-month sojourn into marriage.

My contributions to household expenses were meager during that first year. I taught oil painting and wax work in our neighbors' homes. I wrote a column of local chit-chat for the weekly newspaper, adopting the signature of "Country Cousin." My anger and grief became absorbed into caring for Teddy and helping as much as I could with domestic chores. My Mother seemed to thrive under the added stress of grandmotherhood and Pa revelled in his new role.

Then came the three years of my teaching in Syracuse. That meant seeing Teddy only on weekends and during vacations. I practically abondoned him! . . . He became my parents' little boy during those years that I boarded with a family in the city. My salary as a teacher was paltry but sufficient to provide necessities for my fast-growing son and to help my parents in a small way. My purse strings were drawn tight.

And now Medical School at Syracuse University!! Last month when Pa came up with the brilliant idea of buying a house in the city with proceeds from the sale of the Kirkville cottage, I gasped with unbelief and anticipation.

Tomorrow we shall move to the new place on East Fayette Street a short distance from the medical school. There will be room to spare for all of us and the lot itself has space for a good-sized garden in the backyard. Teddy will start school now in the very building where I used to teach last year. And as time passes, he will have many of my old friends as his teachers. Best of all — I can see Teddy, Pa and Mother every day!

The new way of life brings into focus my ignorance concerning money and the management of a mortgage. Pa wants me some-how to assume responsibility for the house. There are laws govern-ing the ownership of property by women. Pa is almost as ignorant as I am. I have been sheltered from the real world for too long. In contemplating my stupidity I read with interest reports on laws governing a woman's right to inherit property in this morning's paper.

MEDICAL SCHOOL

Sept. 6, 1875

At nine o'clock on the dot Chancellor Haven of this University of Syracuse welcomed us, the entering and returning medical stu-dents, explaining that many serious and learned men had worked

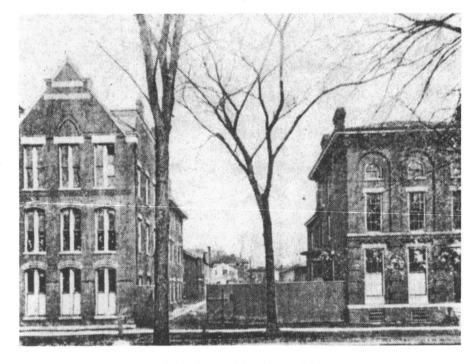

Medical School buildings, 1875.

together to prepare a course of medical study for us reflecting the best science and culture of our time. Ours is a class of fifteen students, the largest class including two women besides myself, to be admitted since the opening of the Medical School in 1872. Most of the men have grown beards, but not one of us women wears a bustle. I know it is difficult to sit on a bustle! And there will be hours of sitting.

The Chancellor emphasized the new philosophy of medical study and clinical experience. Each member of the teaching staff will include in his teaching the history of medicine as it applies to his specialty, ever being alert to new discoveries. The hospitals here will provide us with clinical exposure—a source of teaching which Geneva Medical School lacked.

The faculty tends to be eclectic and open-minded in approach to treatment of disease. The Chancellor then pointed out that this college of medicine, together with those at Harvard and the University of Chicago, takes leadership within the country to require three whole years of study with appropriate examiniations before awarding of medical diplomas.

October 13, 1875

Dr. Didama spoke to us in his lecture today about the communicable diseases including typhoid fever, which have recently caused many deaths in the city. However, it appears that most of the deaths here result from tuberculosis, its etiology still a mystery. In response to the need to provide better control of these diseases as well as measles, whooping cough, smallpox and diphtheria, it has been proposed that there be formed a Board of Health as there is a Board of Education. Just as there is a Commissioner of Education, there shall be a Commissioner of Health to oversee the prevention and control of disease in this city. (I remember my conversation with Dr. VanDuyn last summer in the Pest House about these very same matters.)

Dr. Didama reminded us that it was not long ago that jaundice, for instance, was treated with frequent dosages of a powder concocted from salts of earthworm, hog's lice, skin of hen's gizzard, ground toads and geese's feet! When death occurred, inevitably it was the doctor who explained to the family that there had been a visitation of Divine Providence — Diving Providence being the Angel of Death.

When only ten years ago there had been a serious outbreak of cholera here, action was taken to effect improvement of sanitary conditions in the area. There was drainage of swamp land and investigation into a better source of drinking water as well as a plan for enlarging the so-called Pest House by initiating the "cottage method" so that only patients with similar diagnosis would

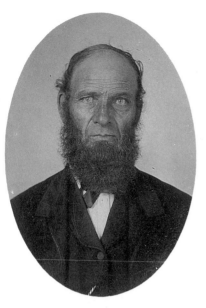

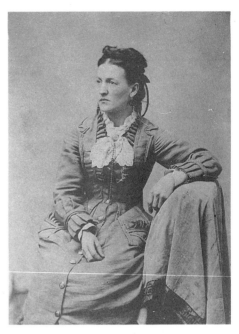

Randolph Lamb, Millie's father, at the time she entered Medical School.

Millie as she began Medical School at Syracuse University, 1875.

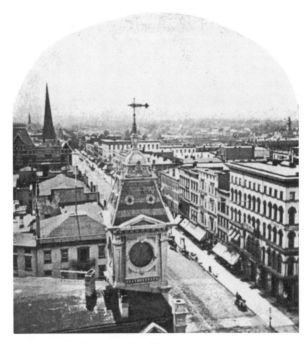

South view of Salina Street in 1875.
(Source: *Syracuse and Its Environs*, Franklin H. Chase)

be cared for in each isolated facility. No visitors would be allowed. It was reported that four members of the County Medical Society had been sued for "false imprisonment of a patient" there within recent months. As a result, members of the County Society spoke in defense of their colleagues publicly and through the City Council of Hygiene explaining the need for quarantine of patients with communicable diseases such as typhoid fever, scarlet fever, some types of pneumonia, cholera, diphtheria, measles, especially if home care were impossible or inadequate. Attention was drawn to the effect of the unabated yellow fever epidemic in the south—cause so far unknown. Reports printed daily in our newspapers.

That lecture brought back in horrible detail my own memories of being a patient in the Pest House last summer—the fever, the delirium, the nightmares, the awful fear, the sounds of agony, the smell of death.

"Medical Science," he said in his genial way, "has evolved from knowledge gained from experience over many years—many eons—and cannot be taught by rule. The purpose of the profession is to *maintain* health and to *alleviate* suffering."

"This School is dedicated to the recognition of disease and the cure of that disease *if it is possible*. We welcome well-qualified men as well as women who shall work together as respected professionals in the practice of the art and science of medicine. As you all know, Elizabeth Blackwell, who was the first woman to receive a medical degree in the United States, graduated at the top of her Geneva class. Some of you in seeking excellence, will follow in her footsteps. Some will inevitably fall by the wayside."

Beginning at eight o'clock in the morning every week-day, classes will include, for the first year, Anatomy, Physiology, Histology, Chemistry, and Botony. Eighteen physicians, including the Dean, make up the faculty. My special friend, Dr. VanDuyn is professor of "general, special, and surgical anatomy" and Dr. William Manlius Smith from Manlius will teach Botony and Materia Medica.

I have fully recovered from typhoid fever and once again feel like my old self. I am ready and eager, as my family — Mother, Pa and Teddy — settle in the new house — new for us — on East Fayette Street only three blocks away from the College. Pa is scheduled to take Teddy after his vaccination against smallpox for his first day at my old school. Teddy and Pa are special pals these days.

November 5, 1875

Well, I have survived the first month. The experience has opened my eyes somewhat as to what lies ahead. Since I was never in my life before rediculed by men because of being a female I have been at a loss to respond effectively. My clothing is old — the same that I wore when I was a teacher. I admit it hangs somewhat loosely on me because of the weight I lost last summer. The men I meet on the street seem to be looking for my missing bustle! And of course my shoes are old, worn and low-heeled. Perhaps to them I seem to be poverty-stricken.

I suspect the old-fashioned look of our garments is what has induced my friend and colleague Ellen, to generate the courage to wear long black trousers — instead of street sweeping skirts — with her blouses, tunics or tight-fitting jackets. I presume our best tactic is to retaliate (if that is the word), to the taunts and leers aimed at us, by total disregard as we are walking in public.

Christmas Day

It has been a cold, snowy happy day for Pa and Mother and Teddy and me to be all together. Pa was able to chop down a beautiful Scotch pine tree from the old wood lot at the farm. And Teddy gave me a profile silhouette of himself that his teacher had cut out. An excellent likeness. I shall frame it. My contributions in the gift department were exceedingly small, but we were all together for the entire day!

New Year's Day 1876

Seven of my class stopped in at our house to celebrate last evening and to meet Mother and Pa and Teddy who had more fun than anyone. We played the old music box with the big perforated metal discs and drank hot spiced cider. Mother passed around plate after plate of sugared fried cakes which some of the men had never tasted before. I played my guitar and Bill W. brought his mandolin. We sang and told stories until one o'clock this morning. We felt like old friends and I hated to see them go home. Invisible barriers had broken. Laughter is a powerful antidote to loneliness. Teddy fell asleep in front of the fireplace curled up on the bear rug as if he were a young cub in hibernation for the rest of the winter. Pa finally carried him upstairs and tucked him into his own little bed.

Tomorrow I shall make time to go sliding with him in the park.

February 3, 1876

I attended a lecture at Shakespeare Hall Tuesday evening — the topic being "The Role of Women in Marriage." Mrs. Victoria Woodhull who, it is reported was once nominated by an Equal Rights Party to run for President of the United States, was the speaker. She has become a well-known public figure and along the way has accumulated a somewhat controversial reputation over the years as she drums up defense and rebuttal for Womens Rights. I was eager to hear what she had to say to the Syracuse audience — both men and women.

She was stylishly dressed in purple silk, spoke clearly with self-confidence using excellent diction. Her message was straightforward, leaving no words capable of being misunderstood. She was serious in both tone of voice and demeanor — "There should be no bringing of children into this world except by mothers who want them." She argued against legal marriage because it deprives women of propagation control by extending it to the male partner.

She went on to assure her audience that every negative pressure brought to bear on a pregnant woman can have a negative deleterious effect on the child she carries.

She pointed out that the human race can be improved by scientific propagation in the same manner as fruits, flowers and animals are improved. She endeavored to explain that the misery, vice and crime with which the earth is cursed can be traced to mothers who have unwillingly allowed themselves to become pregnant. "Undesired, improperly cared for children become the criminals, the insane, the miserable members of our society," she said. . . . "Our earth is sin-bestridden and disease cursed," she reminded us as she quoted from a recent article in the Chicago Times.

"As long as woman is not sexually free and fully educated in all matters that pertain to the begetting and rearing of children, our society is doomed." She stressed that women are innately pure and virtuous and that if they are not forced by pecunious need or custom to propagate the earth, they will remain so. She urged mothers to teach their daughters never to marry a man for his wealth or position or for any reason except for love. . . . She spoke on with fervent words, saying that any woman — no matter what her age — should never marry a man for a motive other than love. If she does so, she is no better than the woman who sells herself promiscuously. "Men must know," she said, "that the inauguration of Woodhull Theories will deprive them of the women who are now in sexual servitude to them."

"Even with this knowledge men persist in proving their superiority and power by abusing women. If a woman chooses marriage and willingly takes on the responsibility of raising children, she must equip herself physically and mentally for the task. On the other hand, if she chooses to remain unmarried and childless, she should expect acceptance and respect from men."

There was scattered applause. Obviously I do not agree wholeheartedly with many of Mrs. Woodhull's tenets — yet I do agree with woman's need to be heard in this society.

The Ides of March

Today in Anatomy class I very nearly lost both my temper and my sense of humor. During the past few weeks I have become initmately acquainted with "Nick," my cadaver.

I have become almost fond of him in a gruesome sort of way. We have all finished studying certain superficial aspects of anatomy and were prepared today to begin dissection of the genito-urinary system.

Lately I have withstood denigrating remarks and attracted the brunt of considerable male humor, most of which I have tended to ignore. I admit though that there have been a few instances when I have hurled back retorts with as decent English as I can muster. It's a challenge.

The overall aura and odor of the place does not give me confidence in myself. I must make a conscious effort to concentrate in order to overcome a frequent sensation of faintness—sometimes even nausea. The dizziness at times makes me unsure of what I am supposed to be observing.

This morning as I took up my scalpel to make the initial incision into Nick's bladder I was mildly conscious of an unusual hush in the room. Suddenly Nick and I seemed to be the center of attention. I gritted my teeth and made a vigorous cut. Out poured a cloud of ill-smelling vapor like an evil genie curling in a continuous spiral above Nick's dried bones and wizened remains. Deep throated guffaws from my fellows.

It developed that the previous evening the lads had spent valuable time inflating Nick's bladder with pipe smoke. All associated valves and blowholes in that portion of his anatomy had been carefully sutured so that they held securely even after that first prick of my scalpel. It seemed to take me a long moment to regain composure. — I laughed and the boys laughed with me.

Except for sharp words of displeasure and admonition from our much loved unsmiling Professor the morning proceeded without further disruption. Actually I probably owe my "friends" gratitude. The male genito-urinary system will remain clearly etched within my memory forever.

April 14, 1876

Today, my birthday, begins a new decade. I am thirty years old, about to begin studying for final examinations after the first year in medical school. In more ways that I can count I am responsible for my seven-year-old son and both my parents. I would not admit it to another human being, but today I feel overwhelemed, frightened, weary, discouraged. How did I ever have the timerity to begin to study again? I had no conception of the interruptions facing me as I opened that Anatomy Book. I could not have imagined the effect of being taunted, mocked, disparaged. Some of the jabs into my psyche have not yet healed and I know there will always be scars. In spite of the hours of study I seem to have lost confidence in myself.

The birthday cake with its chocolate icing Mother had so lovingly made for me only made me want to weep.

It brought into focus many past childhood birthdays when all future seemed bursting with springtime and sunshine. How does a doctor cure himself—especially if that doctor is one who wears skirts and actually revels in the challenge of being a woman? My "disease" is depression—of heart, soul, intellect.

May 1, 1876

I went to church on Sunday with Mother and Pa. For a change my attention was rivited on the minister's words as he spoke about the human meaning of Ecclesiastes Chapter 3 today. Previously I had thought that I should be at home studying for the final examinations which are coming all too soon. That day the Pastor's words seemed to have a personal message directed toward me.

"To every thing there is a season: A time to be born, a time to
die: a time to plant and a time to reap; a time to laugh and a
time to weep; a time to mourn and a time to dance; a time to
embrace and a time to refrain from embracing; a time to
gather and a time to cast away; a time to gain and a time to
lose; a time to keep silence and a time to speak; a time to love
and a time to hate; a time for war and a time for peace."

Right now I feel as if I can add a few words to Ecclesiastes as a
result of living through the past year.

"A time to lose and a time to win;
A time to think and a time to act;
A time to forget and a time to remember;
A time to run, a time to rest;
A time to doubt, a time to pray;
A time for pain, a time for healing;
A time to give, a time to receive;
A time to be alone, a time to join hands;
A time for sunshine, a time for storm;
A time to fear and a time to dare."

At this moment I feel that it is time for me to weave the book of
knowledge I have gained into solid, workable wisdom!!! — Wisdom
that may help to give respite to my own very personal painful
"dis-ease."

May 7, 1876

Last night I had a puzzling dream. I was alone in a windowless,
constricted room. I was looking through the lens of a powerful
magnifying glass. I was watching the fertilization of an egg—
Nature's creative genius at work. I was spying. Suddenly I was
conscious of enlightenment—a dramatization of the beauty of
this beginning of life—life so insignificantly tiny that it could not
have been seen by the naked eye. It was only through this powerful lens that I was witnessing a miracle. As suddenly as the micro-

scopic apparition had appeared, there was gray darkness in the room. I was being enveloped in cold slime. There was movement around me. Vague distorted figures of what I had seen through the lens seemed to be floating around me. They were growing in a ghastly fashion and wrapping themselves about my legs and arms like snakes. Bloated portions of dissociated human organs slid along my face, my neck, up and down my legs. I shuddered and awoke in terror. It was impossible for me to sleep again. What was the significance — the hidden meaning of that dream?

I dressed, went into the back garden, watched the sun rise. A dog barked. The milkman's horse's hoofs clomped down the street and stopped at our house. I could hear the clink of the glass bottles. The old clock in the dining room struck six times. Two exams had been scheduled for that day.

And now it is two weeks later. . . . Utter relief. All examinations passed!

June 6, 1876

The C. family from Manlius want Mother and Pa to stay with them on their farm in July. It will give them a renewed lease on life to be with their old friends again away from the city. I have arranged to send Teddy to Mary G. in the country to visit for awhile. She has a boy about Ted's age. I'll see how he reacts to being away from home. Occasionally I can go out to get a lay of the land and a first-hand look at how he is adapting to being away from home and all of us.

I plan to spend as much time as I can this summer finding out how the City works. I'll talk with the Commissioner of Health, the director of Nurses at the Good Shepherd Hospital and the matron at the Orphans Asylum. And I want to visit the Feeble Minded Institution and talk with Dr. W. there. I am curious about what happens to unfortunate women, girls and children. I'll keep a careful record of what I observe—should be valuable for later on.

Also I want to see how women at the Old Ladies' Home* get along with one another and how the Directress manages to keep peace among the more obstreperous ladies. There and at the Poor House. I think that there the inmates are chiefly men—old men. I understand that some of our cadavers come from there.

Pastor H. told me that there are plans afoot by the women of the Unitarian church to start a Female Employment Society and that they are considering establishing a Day Nursery at the Church for the benefit of working mothers and their young children from all quarters of the city.

Here is a letter just now delivered to me from Teddy—August 29, 1876.

Back at the old Manlius Farm

Dear Mama,

Joe, my loud rooster, don't come into the woods anymore. I leave my coop door open. I am so full of peaches I can't lean over. I am well and so is Grandpa. I am not homesick now Not a bit. Grandma and Uncle Henry have gone riding. I cride a little after you left me. But Grandpa laid down beside me and then I stopped. I fele good now. They is good peaches in the orchard. I wish you was here to have supper with us. I made a box to put special stones in. Mrs. Cook said she saw you and that you looked well. I was glad of it. Please rite me soon. I guess Uncle Henry and Grandma are going to the fair and I wish you could go too. I got almost sick of eating apples and so many peaches. When Grandma and I went to the barn Grandma spoke to a boy in a wagon that was going down the road. When they got past Doctor Phillips house the horse ran away. Might be he got hurt bad. Goodby.

From your Teddy

* Millie would never have guessed that many years later when she was on the Board of Directors for the "Home" that she would take her three granddaughters to call on "the ladies" there to distribute books and magazines and to perform for an hour as "little girls reciting poetry."

The morning I visited the Feebleminded Institute, it was with surprise I noted that some people appeared to me to be normal. Of course there were others in another section of the builidng whose behavior, to say the least, was strange. One woman who was almost naked, sat alone carefully pulling out her graying hairs—one by one—inspecting each hair over its entire length before dropping it onto the floor. No change of expression on her doughy face or glassy eyes. Another young woman grim-faced and tense stood in place see-sawing her entire body back and forth—dark eyes angry and darting. In one corner of the ward, squatting on the floor with their legs drawn up to their chests, two young girls were intentionally indelicately exposing themselves. And further down the ward sat a young man biting his nails and staring at an open book on his lap without turning a page. Not one of the patients paid any attention to me as a strange visitor in the long "violent ward."

After an hour of being conducted through the hospital by the Matron, I kept my appointment with Dr. W. who welcomed me in his office. Seemed pleased that I as a "young" medical student had come to visit the Institute. He explained that all the nurses and attendants have had special training before they come to work here.

All attendants are taught to be kind in their treatment of the patients and at the same time to be constantly alert for sudden changes in mood which often result in physical violence that may be difficult to control.

The staff members are instructed in ways to protect themselves as well as other patients if and when such outbreaks may occur. The doors, as well as the barred windows, are kept locked at all times. Only the doctors and nurses have keys and the head nurse is charged with giving all medications which are kept in a locked cabinet.

I was impressed with recent changes toward the mentally deranged. Dr. Wilbur assured me that some patients are able to return to their homes and families. I asked him about the care of maternity patients who become irrational following the birth of babies. He told me that he has had some patients admitted who have become so depressed that they actually disregard a newborn child. Not only could a new mother at home deny care to her baby, but often she might completely ignore other members of the household, paying no attention to customary domestic duties. Such patients, he told me, during the depth of their depression could harm themselves or attempt suicide.

And then he told me that all physicians who practice obstetrics should follow through in caring for a mother who has lost a baby. Grief is intense, all-encompassing depression.

Doctors and care-givers, he assured me, should realize that parental hopes for nurturing and raising a child can be suddenly blasted. Breasts that were overflowing become swollen and painful, nipples oozing—no babe to suckle. A cradle empty, a grave filled. The mother, and father too, need a source of human compassion.

"You, the physician," he said, "can give extraordinary consolation. Too many doctors actually abandon a family at a time when they are most needed." I had not thought before of this extended function of a family physician. Perhaps as a woman I am better able to assume the role of hope-giver. I hadn't thought before of that aspect of being the kind of doctor I want to be, especially when my patient faces Death . . . Death in any one of its many guises.

Sept. 1, 1876

The second year of Medical School is about to begin. There will be a continuation of the study of Anatomy and Chemistry. In addition there will be much time spent on Materia Medica coordinating it with last year's knowledge of Botony. The afternoons will be devoted to Clinical Medicine and Clinical Surgery. That means seeing patients in the hospital and the clinics with the older doctors—our mentors—Dr. Frederick Hyde and Dr. Henry

College of Medicine.

SYRACUSE UNIVERSITY.

FACULTY.

JOHN TOWLER, M. D., Professor of Chemistry and Toxicology.
FREDERICK HYDE, M. D., Professor of Principles and Practice of Surgery.
HENRY D. DIDAMA, M. D., Professor of Practice and Clinical Medicine.
NELSON NIVISON, M. D., Professor of Physiology, Pathology and Hygiene.
JOHN VANDUYN, M. D., Professor of General, Special and Surgical Anatomy.
EDWARD B. STEVENS, M. D., Professor of Materia Medica and Therapeutics.
CHARLES E. RIDER, M. D. Professor of Ophthalmology and Diseases of the Ear.
HARVEY B. WILBUR, M. D., Lecturer on Insanity.
WILFRED W. PORTER, M. D., Professor of Obstetrics and Diseases of Women.
WILLIAM T. PLANT, M. D., Professor of Clinical and Forensic Medicine.

ROGER W. PEASE, M. D., Professor of Operative and Clinical Surgery.
ALFRED MERCER, M. D., Professor of Minor and Clinical Surgery.
J. OTIS BURT, M. D., Professor of Medical Chemistry and Dermatology.
MILES G. HYDE, M. D., Adjunct Professor of Anatomy.
WM. MANLIUS SMITH, M. D., Professor of Botany and Adjunct Professor of Mat. Med.

J. W. KNAPP, M. D., Demonstrator of Anatomy.
DAVID M. TOTMAN, M. D., Instructor in Physiology.
BRACE W. LOOMIS, M. D., Instructor in Chemistry.

This Year ends Wednesday, June 27th.

Next Year begins Thursday, October 4th.

Students of the Regular Course are required to take the studies, and those only, of the years to which they belong.

SESSION 1876-77.

First Year—Second Term.

Hour	Monday.	Tuesday.	Wednesday.	Thursday.	Friday.
8.30	Anatomy. L.	Anatomy. L.	Histology.	Anatomy. R.	Anatomy. L.
9.30	Physiology.	Physiology.		Physiology.	Physiology.
10.30	Chemistry. L.	Laboratory.	Laboratory.	Laboratory.	Chemistry. R.
2	Practical Anatomy.	Botany.	Practical Anatomy.	Practical Anatomy.	Botany.

Second Year—Second Term.

Hour	Monday.	Tuesday.	Wednesday.	Thursday.	Friday.
8.30	Anatomy. L.	Anatomy. L.		Anatomy. R.	Anatomy. L.
9.30	Physiology.	Physiology.	Pathology.	Physiology.	Physiology.
10.30	Mat. Medica.	Surgery. L.	Chemistry. L.	Mat. Medica.	Mat. Medica.
2	Pr. and Prac. L.	Surgery. R.	Pr. and Prac. R.	Laboratory.	Pr. and Prac. L.
3	Clinical Surgery.	Clinical Medicine.	Clinical Surgery.	Clinical Medicine.	Surgery. L.

Third Year—Second Term.

Hour	Monday.	Tuesday.	Wednesday.	Thursday.	Friday.
10.30	Mat. Medica.			Mat. Medica.	Mat. Medica.
11.30	Obstetrics. L.	Forensic Med.	Obstetrics. L.	Insanity.	Obstetrics. R
2	Pr. and Prac. L.	Surgery. R.	Pr. and Prac. R.	Ophthalmol.*	Pr. and Prac. L.
3	Clinical Surgery.	Clinical Medicine.	Clinical Surgery.	Clinical Medicine.	Surgery. L.

*Until May 1st.

Copy of Millie's Medical School curriculum, 1876-77.

Didama. And Dr. John VanDuyn will be professor of Surgical Anatomy. There will be even less time for me to be with Teddy, but I still count on the week-ends. A convocation is planned to welcome us back as an entire group and to announce changes for the coming year. The Dean has a refreshing sense of humor which I am coming to appreciate.

Next year, our senior year, we will be studying Obstetrics and Gynecology, finally being given the opportunity to deliver some babies. I look forward to that experience. We'll also be delving into insanity and the legal aspects of Medicine, called Forensic Medicine. Otherwise our schedule looks like more of the same work that we are doing this year. Murder!

Mother seems to be skeptical about the influence of some of Teddy's new friends on him. She is not used to the ways of small city boys. No barn chores to attend to and somehow Teddy is no longer as cuddlable as he used to be. As his circle of playmates expands his explorations beyond our house and the schoolyard overspreads a wider and wider circumference. Mother has less control of him and fears the dangers lurking in the city might harm him.

I must find more time (what an elusive, fleeting substance time is!) to be with him, to talk with him. Except for tucking him into bed at night and saying prayers with him, I feel sometimes as if he is growing up a stranger to me. And I should set up a special time to speak with his teacher this year—a new one whom I never met before. She probably doesn't know that I leave the house as he wakes up and don't return until after he has had his supper. What would I ever do without Mother and Pa?

The Circus is coming to town next week. I think Pa would like to take him to see it and to watch the parade beforehand, and I would like to hear the piping of the calliope afterward. And before the weather gets too blowy and cold I would like to take him on a steamboat ride around Onondaga Lake. There might be a band concert on board!

Sept. 15, 1876

I have decided to write Uncle William in New Haven to ask him if he will help me put together a short history of his family. Teddy has already begun to ask me questions about his Father. The answers to my queries addressed to William will be for my own benefit too. Edward and I had not known each other long enough for me to learn much about his story-telling Father John and his spinning and weaving Mother Mary MacPherson with the auburn hair. William will remember I am sure, with some sadness, when eight-and-a-half months pregnant, I made my precipitous departure from his Greene Street house in New Haven.

Since Edward was the last to leave his family, I know he must have felt pangs of guilt more than once. I too was brought up on a farm and know only too well about the hard work, the long hours between sunrise and darkness, the harvest risks, the scarcity of money. I want Teddy to know about his Father's early years of growing up in that big family of twelve children — Dann children. Now and then I presume he resents being the only child in our family.

October 3, 1876

Uncle William did send me several pages of carefully written information concerning his family, including a geneology going back to 1690 at the time of Prince William of Orange when he, later to be known as King William III, crossed the English Channel from the Netherlands with a well-trained army, including three brothers by the name of Dann — our first identifiable ancestors. One of those brothers, a soldier called John, survived the Battle of the Boyne and after the war settled in the north of Ireland with his Irish wife and children. That man was Teddy's ancestor.

Uncle William wrote in his letter dated October 1 to me:

"My main business for the day when I was twelve was to pick up stones from the meadow and pile them in heaps. Sometimes my back ached so that I could hardly stoop down to pick up the heavy rocks. After 5 o'clock milking I drove the cows back to their pasture for the night. My fingers got stiff and sore. Tears often blinded my eyes. Sometimes I had conversations with imaginary people, sang hymns and old Irish ballads to myself. On Saturday nights I walked the four miles back to our house after I had finished churning butter and mending the broken fences. I read books whenever I could, but I liked best to tell stories that I made up, to Edward.

"Our oldest brother, Jonathan, rebelled against our father's discipline and the work he had to do. Father always expected that he would become a farmer but Jonathan loved books, and music and oratory. His defiance within the family opened an unexpected roadway leading away from farm life and paved new directions for the rest of us—his younger brothers.

"Father used to say that he had no money to give us as a financial start in life; all he could do was to provide us with the best education he could and then to let us go—if go we must at eighteen years of age.

"If he had given each of us a thousand dollars it could not have been a more generous gift. We gained independence, self-respect, courage and self-reliance. In the wildest flight of our imaginations we would hardly have dared to picture that now the carriages from our own New Haven factory are in use from Maine to California, even in Mexico, South America, Australia and South Africa. Since the Civil War, the folding chairs which brother John invented are now much in demand in many civilized countries of the world and are used on every steamer that crosses the ocean. We prize one photograph of General Ulysses S. Grant standing beside one of our chairs in front of his tent during the Civil War.

"The old rural Hillsboro Schoolhouse was the real center of our lives. It was church and library as well as school all-year-round.

"Every fall new and used books somehow arrived at the school library. Our minds were steeped in Plutarch's Lives, world history, travel to all points of the compass, poetry and tales of adventure.

"Within the primeval forest which was the main part of our 140-acre farm, north of Oneida Lake, many wild animals lived and roamed. We often saw brown bears, deer, foxes, squirrels, chipmunks and rabbits. And the woods were full of birds of all sorts—from owls to bluebirds.

"I can tell you, Millie, that none of our large family—including Edward—lacked for excitement or love as we grew up."

October 15, 1876

Ted and I did go a-sailing and there was a band concert playing at one of the picnic groves, along the shore of Onondaga Lake on a warm September Sunday afternoon. Ted was right up there with the players fascinated by the different instruments, especially the bassoon! And before we left he had two rides on the merry-go-round. We laughed and talked nonsense and had a wonderful time. The next time I would like to take him in a canoe and teach him to paddle. He loves to come to the lake with Bill to fish from the shore. One of these days he will want to catch a ride on a sailboat to try his luck at catching pike. At least I can feel assured that he knows how to swim and manage himself in the water.

Nov. 15, 1876

This morning Dr. Didama lectured about the recent epidemic of Smallpox in this city.

Some blame has been placed on the landing in this city of certain infected persons from the Erie Canal boats. Vaccination should be mandatory, he said. Not only just for the children being admitted to school! And then he talked about Typhoid Fever and the accepted treatment today. Even now the challenge to save these patients goes on. There are many deaths. How naive I was back in those New Haven days when Edward was so very sick! Because of my lack of knowledge I may have unaccountably

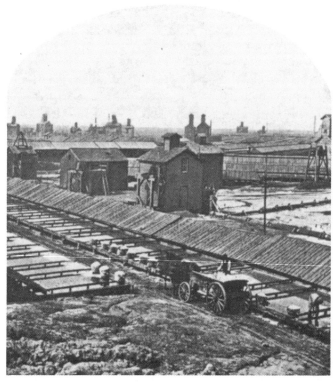

Salt vats for evaporation and nearby housing for workers' families, 1875.

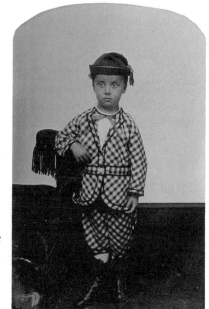

Tintype of Teddy at the age of six, 1875.

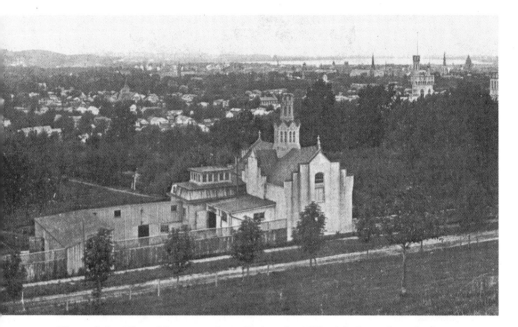

View of the City of Syracuse from University Hill with Onondaga Lake in the background, 1875.

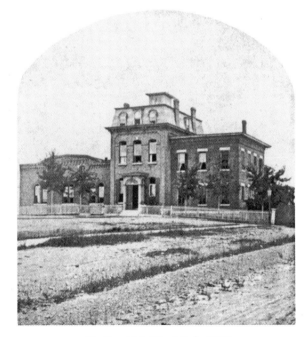

St. Joseph's Hospital, 1875.

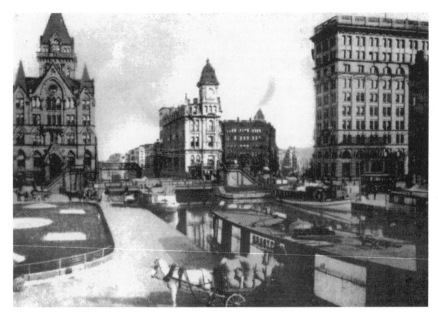

Packet Dock, Erie Canal in 1876.
(Courtesy of The Erie Canal Museum)

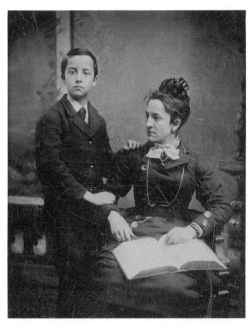

Millie with her son on his ninth birthday,
February 7, 1878.

contributed to the complications of his disease and even to his death. Horrible thought.

Dec. 20, 1876

Henry has written that he will be coming east to spend Christmas with us. Mother has been cleaning, cooking, sewing and Pa has conjured up at least ten chores he needs help with around the house. It will be like old times to have Henry drag in a Christmas tree and help to trim it. I have been making a few small gifts to do up and put underneath the Scotch pine tree. We shall have two weeks of vacation. I am looking forward to some extra sleep myself. This term has been extraordinarily demanding. Some days I feel bewildered!

Feb. 7, 1877

Today, February 7, 1877, is Teddy's eighth birthday. I wish his Father could see him. He is tall for his age, has features much like his father's—not at all like mine, even when I was a child. He is doing well in school, according to Miss B., but I think if he had his druthers he would be out playing in the snow. His Grandfather has found a little puppy to give him as a present today. He has some collie blood in him and is a beautiful little tri-color mutt with four white feet and a white-tipped tail. It will be good for Ted to have a dog of his own to care for and to love. And it will be up to him to choose a name for him. I have fixed up a wicker basket as a bed. Supposedly he has been paper-trained, but I, for one, wouldn't count on it. I think Ted will want to keep him in his room at night. Of course he will!

June 20, 1877

Wild strawberries with our cereal this morning. Teddy and Bill picked them from a nearby field. Delicious essence reminds me of the farm. Those two enterprising young'uns are now out ringing neighbors' doorbells, taking orders for the small newspaper they have plans for printing themselves this summer. Now and then they discover a kind soul willing to buy an ad!

These adventures of theirs please me more than the hair-raising story Teddy told us at supper last night. The two boys, when workmen were away from the building site at lunchtime, climbed a tall ladder inside the new St. Mary's Catholic Church—to the top of the apse where they each confessed they had carved their initials onto a supporting beam.

Another time Teddy admitted that he had set off a false alarm to the fire department in order to create a little excitement. The clanging of the bells, the sounding of the sirens and the racing hoofs of the horses promoted more thrills to that boy of mine than the most adventuresome story in his bookcase. If I had time, I might worry about him.

Years ago when we lived with his grandparents in Kirkville, I remember clearly watching my Mother as she rocked him in the old Boston chair by the kitchen window. It was winter time. Frost had etched itself on the inside of the old windowpane. He looked up at her sleepily as she crooned,

> "Wonderful pictures—silver white
> Gleam on the windowpanes tonight:
> Stately forests and orchard trees,
> Birds and blossoms and honeybees.
> No one can tell how the pictures grew—
> Wonderful pictures—silver and white."

My Mother told me that on a cold frosty morning she used often in the wintertime to sing the same song to her children in the one-room schoolhouse where she was once a country school teacher.

August 3, 1877

There was a disgusting article in the *Courier* today. Headlines:

"A PLAGUE AMONG US . . . SECRETS OF THE DISSECTING
ROOM REVEALED!"

The account went on to describe festering bodies at the Syracuse University Medical College. "A nauseous stench pervades the
atmosphere. Residents living near the college must close their
windows although the temperature today was predicted to be in
the 90's. Just before or after a rainstorm the effluvia is most
offensive because of the high humidity. Some persons have suggested that the odor is coming from the sewer running beneath
Fayette St. Several residents, it is reported, have vacated their
homes."

A *Courier* reporter in an attempt to discover the cause and
possible origin of the stench "pinpointed the small two-story brick
building just east of the main medical school building. He discovered a door on the south side of the structure unbolted."

He "entered the building, mounted the stairs, opened another
door on the second floor leading to a large room. On top of a
table in the center of the room lay a human body in an advanced
state of decomposition. One leg stuck out at the side of the table.
The trunk, head and arms had been mutilated and disfigured.
The body was alive with maggots, the fetid odor indescirbable."

A statement signed by the Medical School Dean and members
of the Faculty was published the next day in the Syracuse *Journal*.
I quote it in its entirety:

> "There is nothing remarkable noted in the history of
> American Journalism which prohibits the publication of sensa-
> tional articles. Startling revelations have been made, horrible
> and monstrous wickedness brought to light.
>
> "Such an exploit has been attempted by the *Courier News*.
> Its reporter has made an enterprising success, but the article
> bares a character of reckless and disengenuous bravado intend-
> ing to stimulate the passions of the ignorant, minister to a mor-
> bid, vulgar curiosity in order to sell papers.
>
> "It happens that the Medical School has been closed for over
> a month. The student who was in charge of the building has

gone home for his vacation, having left the building entirely
locked, the dissection room clean and the specimens in their
proper places. It now appears that the building has been
broken into, specimens removed from the solutions in which
they were kept. Someone has scattered them about the room
and has subsequently invited the public to view "the diabolical
manner with which our faculty were outraging common de-
cency."

"Dissection rooms are just as essential to a medical college as
a recitation room is to a school. No physician can be skillful in
his profession or worth a straw in his community without knowledge of anatomy. Of necessity, a dissection room is not dedicated to non-professional visitors."

Within two days after those words were printed the Dean of the
School and all the faculty signed an authenic denial of the accu-
sation which was published in BOTH newspapers. The stench has
completely subsided.

April 10, 1878

I was lucky to be called by our professor of obstetrics to accompany him last night to the Salt Flats shack of one of our charity
patients already in labor. She was surrounded by a bevy of neighbor women. Each one had a different old wives bit of advice as
the paitent continued to call loudly on God for help. I managed
to disperse most of the visitors, designating only one to boil water
and find clean towels for our use. A child's face appeared from
behind a curtain—a boy of about ten. I enlisted his enterprising
assistance to catch and dispose of a parade of cockroaches as they
marched across the wall near the patient's bed.

Labor proceeded normally and with Dr. K's encouragement I
attended to the last moments of birth—a well-formed male child
with a lusty cry. I shall not forget the quiet joy I felt at that time—
my first delivery. I barely noticed the persistent parade of cockroaches as they raced toward a crack in the wall.

May 15, 1878

I gathered my courage a week after my visit to the Syracuse
Orphans' Asylum in their new building on East Genesee Street to
take a more careful look at our city. Although the Asylum was
scrupulously clean, the children militarily organized, seemingly
well-fed and healthy—still I have been distressed. I spoke with the
Matron about over-all planning for the childrens' future. Of
course some children are placed there temporarily during times of
family crises, some are orphans with one or both parents dead,
but the majority remain abandoned in the institution for years
unless adoption intervenes. When a girl becomes the age of sixteen she may be hired as domestic help in a private home and boys
may be placed into factory jobs or taught a trade. Some schooling
is provided, but there is obvious lack of a home-like atmosphere
to encourage study or reading. Comfortable chairs are few and
far between. Books are scarce. In one room there are puzzles and
games provided with tables and chairs appropriate for various
ages. Lighting is poor. In the dormitories, beds are lined up and
segregated according to gender and age of the occupants. Meals
are served in a huge dining room. Clean clothing is provided and
volunteer seamstresses do the mending.

Outdoor play is confined to a fenced-in yard. Annual outings
are provided by members of the Board of Directors or the Ladies'
Auxiliary. Work is assigned as chores to the children. However,
the heavy tasks and cooking are done by a hired staff of workers.
There seems to be a generous community support. Foodstuff is
brought in regularly by friends and provided copiously especially
during the summer and autumn months, under the direction of
various churches in the community.

In spite of disease epidemics in the city, the Asylum children
have survived with only a few deaths. If a child becomes seriously
ill, he is isolated from the others. As the Matron accompanied me
through the building I heard no sounds of wailing or crying, no
signs of uncontrolled fighting. Neither did I hear laughter. Obvi-

ously the discipline is strict. The "orphans" are kept off the street and their needs for shelter, food and clothing are provided. Sunday School may give the children an introduction to some Bible stories, but I could feel what the children must have felt — starvation for love.

I had read in the paper that Mayor George Belden who was a member of the Board of Directors of the Asylum, had offered his expansive yard and home on James Street as site for a day-long special event for the children. There had been a picnic prepared and served by his wife and ladies of the church. There had been supervised races, games and entertainment. It was also reported that all inmates had been transported in coaches with discipline provided by the Asylum directors.

I was inspired to write a letter to the Mayor, explaining my interest in the new Orphans' Asylum. He responded by inviting me to meet him in his office for a 10-minute appointment the following Tuesday afternoon.

Being in an obviously affable mood he shook hands with me and offered a chair opposite his desk. I introduced myself as a senior medical student planning to practice in the city. I then explained that having once been a teacher in the public school system of Syracuse I was particularly interested in education of the orphans as well as gaining a better understanding of the legal aspects of adoption. He promised to provide me with information in written form on both topics saying that he appreciated my concerns.*

As I rose to leave I commended him on his determination to press for obtaining Skaneateles Lake as the new source of pure water for the city, since my interest too is disease prevention. A grin spread over his face as he grasped my hand.

---

* Little did either Mayor Belden or Millie realize at that time, the influence she was privileged to exert many years later in moving the Home for Orphans to the outskirts of the city, reconstructed as separate "cottages" with a "father" and a "mother" in charge during her term on the Board.

June 30, 1878

Three long years of study for me have finally ended! Last night I graduated with a Doctor of Medicine degree. Mother, Pa and Teddy were there to watch me in my black mortar board and gown, as I received my parchment diploma from Dean Hyde — one of fourteen graduates.

The program was lengthy and impressive at the Wieting Opera House before a large audience. I was surprised so many people attended. The stage was outrageously decorated with huge vases of flowers. There we were seated with the Chancellor of the University and all our faculty. Drescher's orchestra played and Rev. Thurber began the ceremonies with a prayer — he must have known I and the other two women in the class needed to be prayed for! The doctor from Elmira who gave the address spoke chiefly about reform in medical education.

By the time our worthy professors had spoken and a benediction pronounced Teddy had fallen asleep. Pa and Mother took him home while my good friends and I walked in procession to the Vanderbilt House where an excellent supper awaited us. More speeches and special words in verse to the "Lady Members of the Profession" (stupid and unnecessary I thought). In general we applauded the wit and humor of those who toasted us. By midnight I was utterly exhausted.

As I lay in bed afterward I thought of my Edward and how I miss him. Yet if there had been no typhoid fever to claim his life and almost to have claimed mine there would have been no M.D. after my name tonight.

A few days after my graduation, we were having Sunday dinner together — Pa, Mother, Teddy and I. Abruptly Pa excused himself, disappeared for a few moments, reappeared with a small white box tied with a gold cord. "Mother and I," he said quite solemnly, "have a present for you." It was a beautiful gold watch attached to a long gold chain to circle around my neck or suspend

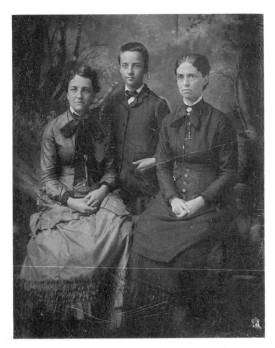

Millie with Teddy and her mother at her graduation.

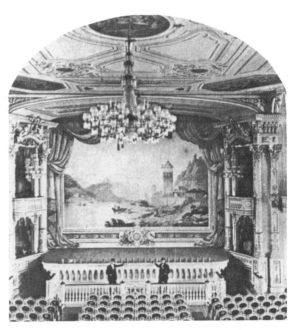

Wieting Opera House auditorium, site of Millie's graduation, June 1878.
(Source: *Syracuse and Its Environs*, Franklin H. Chase)

from a gold pin over my heart. They had purchased it at the finest jewelry store in the city with their sparse savings. "Notice the second hand," Mother added, "and the engraving on the back A.E.D. for our Amelia Eunice. You can count a pulse now without borrowing your Pa's big old watch." Somehow I could not control the tears that kept filling my eyes.

July 5, 1878

Temporarily we have reorganized the parlor of the house on East Fayette Street to be the waiting room of my OFFICE. The dining room will become the examining room with the sturdy examining table old Fred McC. fashioned for me. And I have taken the old dresser from my room to hold my instruments and bottles of medicines. There too will be the brass scales, the magnifying glass, test tubes and measuring cylinders. The old grandfather clock with its striking chimes still stands in the corner to remind me that a new day begins. A table in the kitchen will be transformed into my "laboratory" with the stove to function for boiling instruments. I am ready for action. And there will be a few toys for children — blocks, a wooden train, a few washable animals and books too.

Best of all on the front porch just to the right of the entrance has been placed a metal plaque embossed with the gold letters

AMELIA E. DANN, M.D.

I have hired a young woman, Annie B., who will help Mother in the kitchen and keep the office and upstairs clean. I have already taught her how to sterilize the instruments on the stove. And today I bought a black leather bag for all the paraphernalia I must carry with me to make a house call.

There is a special rack in the bag for little medicine bottles and plenty of room for my stethoscope, thermometer, tourniquets, syringe and needles, catheters, bandages, adhesive and other first aid items. It does look exceedingly professional and at the same time right now very new — very unused!

July 6, 1878

Today I have had my first patient. I answered the doorbell when it rang. There he stood — a lad of ten years — a nondescript puppy in his arms with a fishline hanging ominously from his left eyelid where the hook had snagged. I put my arm around the trembling boy and ushered him into my sancto-sanctorum, calmed him down a bit and quickly managed to sever the hook as the pup yapped bloody murder. The lad looked up at me, grinned, yanked up his sagging breeches, led his tail-wagging dog to the door and with a backward glance, a wave of his hand and a murmured "Thank-ye Mam," he was off — the pup following close to his master's bare heels.

Well, it's a beginning.

July 15, 1878

Teddy came back home with his Grandfather tonight with an eye-sparkling tale of adventure. The two of them had taken the morning stage coach back to Manlius to visit some friends of Pa's who live near the old farm. Teddy had opened the gate to the pasture. Bonny B. was still there — one of our old-time best milkers. She was now a part of Farmer A.'s growing herd. She had a rope tied around her neck with the cowbell still attached. Ted gave her a handful of alfalfa, patted her jowl as she munched. Somehow he managed then to scramble up onto her back.

In a vain effort to dislodge him Bonny Belle took off on a run, circling the pasture, disrupting groups of surprised grazing cattle — the cowbell clanking. Ted held onto the neck rope with all his might calling whoah!! At last, weary from her unaccustomed frolic Bonnie Belle slowed to an amble and Ted slid off her back. The other cattle simply stood still, stared and chewed their cuds.

No lasting harm to beast or boy. Both survived. However,

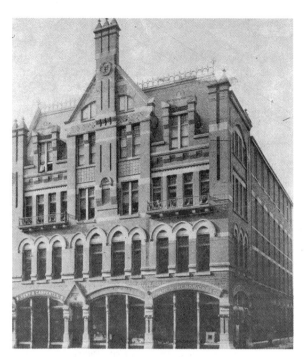

Hendrick's Block in downtown Syracuse, built in 1878. Millie's first downtown office is No. 5.

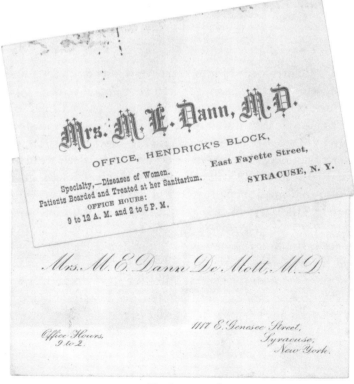

Mrs. M. E. Dann, M.D.

OFFICE, HENDRICK'S BLOCK,

Specialty,—Diseases of Women.
Patients Boarded and Treated at her Sanitarium.

East Fayette Street,

SYRACUSE, N. Y.

OFFICE HOURS:
9 to 12 A. M. and 2 to 5 P. M.

Mrs. M. E. Dann De Mott, M.D.

Office Hours,
9 to 2.

1117 E. Genesee Street,
Syracuse,
New York.

Business cards.

Farmer A. has informed us that Bonnie B. let down not a drop of milk into her pail tonight.

July 25, 1878

Dr. VanDuyn asked me to come to his home on Salina St. to see him last evening after supper. It was the first time I had been in his home or met any of his growing family. A privilege it was — just to sit in his library study. The blue chair he offered me near his desk was velvet covered and comfortable. Sunset rays beamed through the thin curtains at the window. And the new baby cried.

He invited me to make house calls with him as part of my regular schedule. He needs help in doing minor surgery in the home. I can provide another pair of hands. I may also be changing dressings on some of his surgical patients whom I already have met through my work at the hospital. He actually seemed pleased that I "could arrange valuable time to help." I feel honored.

July 30, 1878

Dr. VanDuyn called for me early yesterday morning and off we drove in his Doctor's carriage. First we stopped at the hospital to see three of his post-operative cancer patients and then to make house calls. He introduced me as Dr. Dann — his "associate." Suddenly I was at ease. He is kindly and big-brotherly toward me. He is a well-trained surgeon — trained on the battlefield during the Civil War and a Louisville, Kentucky Medical School graduate. He also told me about his youthful days at Princeton University where he graduated in 1862. He has a sense of humor, pays sharp attention to what a patient says or asks, but wastes no time in unnecessary banter as he works. I like him.

There are fourteen telephones being used in the city so far. If a call comes through the central office for Dr. VanDuyn the operator can locate him simply by referring to a list of designated addresses he has left with her earlier in the day. He has attached to the list an approximate time schedule of the visits he expects to make so that she can send a message to him at any time.

In that way of sleuthing, a worried father located us at the Gray's home on Jefferson St. Ed O'Brian was flushed in the face and out of breath. He knew he had found the doctor when he saw the familiar buggy standing in front of the house with the horse tied to the hitching post. He banged at the door, insisting on seeing the doctor right away. He said his child had been run over by a wagon wheel as the driver was about to deliver ice at the house on the corner. He did not see the boy as he darted into the street. We detoured to the man's home where we found an hysterical mother and a bleeding youngster. Dr. VanDuyn asked to have the kitchen table cleared and a freshly ironed sheet spread over it. His calm, comforting voice soon reassured the parents and with a steady hand he cleansed and disinfected the ugly gash on the boy's forehead, affixing a few stitches. With a promise to return in three days, we were off, as the horse, called Prince, well understood, for the next stop on the doctor's rounds.

August 5, 1878

My neighbors seem frankly curious about "the woman doctor" since the day my shingle was hung by the door. True, the neighbors may become a vanguard of patients when they have need for an available doctor. Mrs. T. from next door brought me a fresh red rose from her garden this afternoon as she welcomed me and my family to the neighborhood. And she smiled. I know that most of the men who have been in practice for years will not be pleased that I have decided to open my office here nor will they be ready to refer women patients to me. In spite of the lack of a red carpet I feel certain that there will be some ladies in this town who will soon come to me for advice and the kind of care I shall be able to give them.

Teddy asked me this morning very seriously, "Mama, when I am sick, can you make me better?" He has been afraid of old Dr.

Brown with the long gray whiskers and bad breath ever since his
last winter's ordeal with the measles.

                                                       Aug. 7, 1878

Mother is determined to maintain our nourishment. They both
— Mother and Pa — boarded the horsecar heading for the Public
Market this morning to replenish our supply of fresh vegetables,
cheese and fruit. They may come back with some sort of meat as
well. Our supply of salt pork hanging in the cellar has been
depleted. More than procuring food, they will relish the talk with
other farmers and their wives who have brought produce to town
today. They revel in comparing prices and quality. Pa will smoke
his pipe, find an old farmer willing to talk about this year's crop
of oats and tobacco. Mother will stop at a bakery booth and com-
pare recipes, find out who is taking jams and jellies and country
pickles next month to the State Fair here. They'll both be coming
home weary and full of stories to tell us.

                                                   September 6, 1878

My Mother's death has come unexpectedly. Our move from the
country to the city has been more arduous for her than I realized.
I know too that the extra work involved in caring for this big
house and her venturesome nine-year-old grandson has taken a
toll on her health. Her heart suddenly gave out after a long day of
activity—Sunday, supposedly the Day of Rest. After the hot walk
from church, she prepared dinner and we all ate together—enjoying much talk, a bit of gossip and laughter.

As she began to clear the table, I heard her gasp and then
quietly moan. She staggered. I helped her to the settee where she
collapsed—pale, blue-lipped and struggling for breath. As I sat
beside her I raised her head against my breast and fanned her.
She looked up at me with fear in her eyes.

Pa and Teddy stood in the dining room doorway like immov-

able statues, terror reflected in their eyes. Mother calmed, re-
laxed a bit as I cradled her in my arms trying to reassure her. She
smiled. Then haltingly she began to repeat the familiar words,
"The Lord — is my shepherd —" In a few fleeting moments she
was gone.

We are all absolutely devastated. The funeral will be here day
after tomorrow afternoon at two o'clock. Burial at the old Manlius cemetery in the family plot.

                                                    Oct. 1, 1878

Last evening I spoke to Pa suggesting that he change his room
to the smaller one that overlooks the garden. He looked through
me—not at me—and seemed mildly agreeable. The room is large
enough to accomodate his single bed and the old oak chest of
drawers he has called his own for many years. There is also plenty
of room for his desk and a comfortable chair; also he wants the
commode with its chamber pot although of course the bathroom
is just around the corner. A picture of his favorite old roan horse
and sleigh could hang on the wall. Mother's tin-type photograph
taken last year with Ted and me in its bamboo frame, would still
be on his dresser along with Mother's silver comb and brush. And
the linen bureau scarf she embroidered.

With Mary's help I moved the furniture while he was out in the
garden this afternoon.

When he came back into the house he shouted, "Amelia, why
have you changed my room? Where is the bed your mother and I
have slept in all these years? Don't you know that what was good
enough for us together is fine for me now! And where is my
Bible?"

Angry tones—the like of which I haven't heard from him since
I was a child.

"I want you should haul it all back just as it was—you hear? As
God is my witness, I mean it!"

I tried to explain to him again that now I have decided to care for a few special patients in the house as if they were in a sanitarium, I need the big front room. Plenty of space there for two beds, two dressers and chairs. At supper he was still adamant —red in the face. And I was tired. He finally agreed to put off making the decision until tomorrow morning.

I brought him a glass of warm milk and a soda cracker at bed time. It seemed to take the hurt out of his eyes. He agreed to try the new room.

November 3, 1878

The experience I had last summer in New York City at the Women's College and Infirmary was indeed valuable to me. There were daily rounds at the hospital—often with Dr. Elizabeth Blackwell herself who had come back for a visit from England. Daily we conferred with patients at the Clinic observing the delivery of babies both at the institution and in slum tenements. I also had the opportunity of assisting in the operating room as well as witnessing surgery and techniques entirely new to me. I attended lectures and had individual conferences with the women professors. The entire staff at the hospital and professors at the college are women— gracious intelligent women.

While I was living in the city, I visited two museums, listened to three outdoor concerts, attended a poetry reading and was invited to Sunday evening gatherings at the homes of three staff members.

February 2, 1879

The time had come—sooner than I realized it would—to talk with Teddy about "birds and bees" and homo sapiens too. This afternoon I found him in my study stretched out in front of the bookcase dedicated to my medical books. He had not heard me enter the room. He was lying on the floor entranced with one of my obstetrical texts. The book was open to a page illustrating in vivid detail the last stage of delivery. The infant's head was stretching the perineum just prior to birth of the child. He looked up at me pale as a ghost, his hand trembling. He slammed the volume shut, tried to replace it on the shelf. "Mother, I didn't know it happened this way!"

I pulled the book out again, sat down beside him on the floor attempting in the simplest words I could find to explain to him the wonderful story of birth. He was an apt listener with questions spilling as I hoped they would. His honest, unembarrassed attitude will lead to more conversations — soon. He told me he was sure Bill and Elmer never talked about these things to their mothers. I told him that oftentimes fathers talked to their sons rather than mothers, but since Ted had no father, it was quite right that he and I should feel free to discuss these matters. I would have much more to tell him. Together we pushed the book back in its place on the library shelf. The ruddy, healthy-boy color once more diffused his face.

And here is a letter from Teddy written July 20, '79 when he was ten:

Dear Mama,

I got up to Utica all right and went up to Mrs. Green's and stayed there awhile. Then she took me to the Dudley house but Mrs. Dudley was not at home. Then we took the train for West Winfield and when we got there we took the stagecoach and it cost me ten cents. And when we got there I thought I wasn't going to like it. No good reason. I am all right now. Mrs. Green got the trunk checked just in time. She asked the baggage man to carry her satchel and he did just as the train was leaving. I ran and got on and the baggage man helped Mrs. Green on.

Things have cost me so far 96 cents. Good by. I hope I see you soon. I really have been away from you long enough. Plenty I think.

                              Your everlasting Frend
                              Edward Howard

P.S. Mrs. Green sends her love and is quite well. Her two

kittens are dead. She wants your picture and mine together.

September 1, 1879

A stylishly dressed young woman sat in my waiting room — a worried far-away look on her face. The high heels she wore necessitated short, mincing steps as she came into the examining room. In answer to my questions, she told me of her recent marriage to a man she had just discovered was drinking so much alcohol — particularly brandy — that she was beginning to fear his rampages. In the bedroom he often became violent and, to punish her for not accepting his husbandly advances, would slap her face, beat her until she wept, pull her breasts and bite her nipples until they bled. She thought her husband was punishing her because she had not become pregnant. — Do men usually act that way, she wondered. In spite of her recitation describing her husband's behavior she said she wanted a child — not just to satisfy her husband. Being a bit nonplussed at that moment I decided the best way to go on with the discussion was to show her an anatomical diagram of the upright female human form. The illustration which I often use, shows a nude drawing — back straight, head erect and well-aligned, breasts small and firm, abdomen flat, arms and legs untensed, feet parallel, toes straight.

She complained further of pain in her abdomen, sick headaches, shortness of breath, constipation and irregular periods. Later as she lay on the examining table, I noted the depressed markings from her corset which etched a design around her waist and onto her abdomen and buttocks.

Now that the corset lacings were released, her bulbous abdomen indicated clearly that her internal organs had been forcibly constricted. Her legs were swollen, her feet mis-shapen, her toes overlapping.

We talked about present-day styles. We talked about the effect of tightly laced corsets on a young woman's torso, the inevitable crowding of stomach, intestines, liver and the constricting pressure on her womb and bladder. She then told me about the purchase of her expensive trousseau and how she wouldn't be able to wear even one of her dresses if she didn't pull in her waist with a proper corset. A complete extravagant waste! I reminded her of her hope to become pregnant—what then would become of her wardrobe? She admitted that the possible need for maternity clothes had not occurred to her!

Our conversation after the examination dealt with a plan to discuss calmly with her husband the problems concerned with bringing a child into the world. I asked that she return to see me after talking over the matter with her husband. We could then deal sensibly with her other queries.

Sept. 1879

I miss the farm—especially at this time of year. I miss its colors, its smells, its integrity. A hayfield is permanently etched in my memory—its oil painting quality of elm trees in the background, the gold of the haystack, the faded blue overalls of the men with their big straw hats, the colorful skirts swirling on the women, the long braids and bright bandanas on the young girls. Brilliant under the late summer sunshine the farm workers' facility in tossing the hay with their pitchforks to the wagon reminds me of a ballet. I find myself searching to find harmony in my own life. From Millie the farm girl, in such a short period of time, I have become Millie the student, Millie the soldier's sister, Millie the school teacher, Millie the bride and housewife, Millie the widow, Millie the mother, a teacher again and now Millie the doctor and bread winner.

My challenge is to develop ability to feel empathy and express sympathy, to give as well as receive enlightenment in a controlled fashion. At times when I am taking a patient's medical history, I sense that in spite of all the information and statistics I have gathered and the physical signs I have noted, still I have missed vital clues. My frustration communicates to the patient. I don't want a patient to lose faith in me. I must sharpen my powers of observation—not only as a doctor, but as a WOMAN doctor.

At times I seem able to gain insight into problems and situations when there is absolute silence, even as I sleep. At other times my strength comes from simply linking a look or touching a patient—her hand, her arm, her shoulder, her forehead.

Perhaps I have been reading too many medical books and journals. I feel the need to take time out again to absorb poetry and philosophy—to reacquaint myself with the poets I have learned to love, with the philosophers I wish I had known.

October 10, 1879

When Janie O. came into the office today complaining of dizziness, aches and pains, I remembered the symptoms I felt a few years ago when I was laid low with typhoid fever. I took her temperature—102 degrees. Her face was flushed. She felt nauseated. When I questioned her, she told me that the family was still using the old farm well behind the outhouse. Her grandmother had died recently after only a week's illness with symptoms similar to Janie's. I am suspicious that the well water may be contaminated. The farm itself is located near a swamp area. I have also determined to make a house call myself to examine the other members of the family and to determine if Janie should be admitted to the hospital (sadly still called the "Pest House"). There are already a growing number of known typhoid cases in the city.

I remember my fear when Dr. VanDuyn checked me into that institution. I was so conscious of the agony Edward had suffered, my total ignorance about the disease, my overpowering grief at the time of his death and the terrifying knowledge after being told of the diagnosis, that I too might die leaving our five-year-old son an orphan. I am forever grateful for the excellent care I received there.

There was an account appearing for February 30, 1880 in the Journal describing Millie's visit to interview the Chief of Police. She had been disturbed by a report that there was a protective philosophy emanating from the Commissioner's office toward the existence of bordellos and prostitution in town.

Millie described the Chief as "gruffly polite," making a half effort to stand when she entered his office. Smelling strongly of cigar stench, the entire place seemed to Millie to be heavy with smoke. When she introduced herself as Doctor Dann, chiefly interested in the diseases of women, the Chief remarked that he had heard of no female doctor in Syracuse who wasn't a quack. On referring to an available list of physicians posted on his desk, he said, "Here there is a *Miller* Dann. Are you that *man?*"

Millie questioned the Chief regarding the matter of arrest of known prostitutes, fully realizing that the city's vice district was centered in the heart of the downtown area near the New York Central depot in well-known hotels, disorderly saloons, and brothels. He admitted that the so-called Red Light-District had existed in the area for many years. "Yes," he added, "especially during the summer months our jail is filled." He acknowledged that with a strong voice of citizen complaint, there were police raids with wholesale driving the women to nearby cities, such as Utica and Rochester, with accompanying police escort. "If a convention is scheduled to meet here," he further admitted, "we know what to expect. Many gentlemen here are ready and willing to put up bail for the ladies."

Before leaving, Millie spoke of the recent spread of venereal disease in town. His retort to her was that she, a woman, could do nothing about that situation: his suggestion was to talk with the docs at the medical school. Dismissing the subject, he seriously informed her that this matter of prostitution is nothing new — it had been going on since before she was born.

As he dismissed her he commented on other problems that concerned his department, such as the public nuisance college boys were becoming on Saturday nights when it wasn't even safe for young children to be on the streets.

March 14, 1880

She walked into my office shoulders squared, eyes vindictive. Annie McB. was concentrating her gall on the unfairness of her fate. Her story spilled: she had come as the oldest of seven children with her parents as recent immigrants from Ireland, having landed in New York City at a point of mass disembarkation for aliens. Her father, discouraged with endless days of inability to find a job, decided to move his family upstate to Syracuse. He hoped for more luck in securing employment in this smaller city where bicycles and typewriters were now being manufactured. He did get a job, but only as a laborer. With family illness came bad times. Scarce money went for drink at the corner saloon.

At the age of 13 Annie left school to work in one of the city's dance halls as a clean-up girl. Proud of being able to bring home a few paltry dollars, she responded with no hesitation to the chance of gathering in more money. Manna from heaven, she thought, for her destitute family when the offer came from the dapper owner of the dance hall to "entertain" the swarm of men who frequented the place at night. With the added enticement of a new red silk dress to wear while she worked at the job, she took her new role seriously. In the meantime, her vista of employment was expanding.

Expanding—to the extent that now as a newly initiated call girl, she had the full-blown rash of recently acquired syphilis. She wondered if she had caught "a case of the chicken pox." She was angry.

Within five minutes she learned not only that she had syphillis but that she was also pregnant. It was a hard way to "grow up." What was "syphilis"? How could she be pregnant? She was really only thirteen. I sent her home to tell her mother and father and made arrangements for her to be admitted to the hospital as a charity patient.

A follow-up report on Annie McB. Her hospital experience ended in a spontaneous abortion. Treatment of her syphilitic infection was begun. Within six weeks she had made up her mind to leave the dance hall and to find a "respectable" job. Appearing at least sixteen, she applied for employment at a local store selling men's furnishings. She was assigned to the necktie department. Having recently acquired the ancient art of coquetry, she utilized her new-found talents as a means of successful selling. One young man about town who often found his way to the necktie counter recognized her developing talents. Within another month, she was sharing his bed—no longer choosing his ties. He was quick to recognize her potential for augmenting his work as the youngest pimp in the city. Her serious life of prostitution had begun.

In the meantime, syphilis and gonorrhea have spread mightily in this town.

May 2, 1880

Dr. VanDuyn stopped in to see me at my office this afternoon. He brought with him a form for me to fill out. It was a printed request addressed to the Onondaga County Medical Society—an application for membership. He encouraged me to fill it out, but with words of warning let me know that he was not entirely optimistic about the outcome. Only one woman has ever been admitted and she has had at least a year of graduate medical study abroad. Do it—do it now, he said. I shall back you.

I know it would be a feather in my female cap to be an active member of the Society. I am sure I could make a positive contribution and at the same time learn a great deal myself. These two years have been an uphill struggle but now many more patients are coming to see me, most of whom have been recommended by other patients. I am convinced that there is a real need for me in this city. So I shall apply with trepidation.

May 10, 1880

Yesterday I was asked to appear before the Governing Board of the Medical Society. One doctor with his thumb tucked under his waistcoat lapel, inquired if I had ever advertised myself as a "specialist." Yes, I had I suppose. There had been an article in the *Courier* reporting that I had returned from studying at the New York infirmary for Women in New York City, the hospital that Elizabeth Blackwell and her sister Emily had established. I was reported to have reopened my new office downtown as a "specialist in the treatment of the diseases of women." The Board rejected me as a member of the County Society.

I then immediately withdrew my application.

Following the letter of rejection from the County Medical Society, Dr. William S. sent me a note. He wrote:

Dear Millie,

When I heard of your request for membership being turned down—at least for the present—I remembered wise words I once read:

'You have no enemies you say?
Alas, my friend, the boast is poor:
He who has mingled in the fray
That the brave endure
Must have made foes! If you have none,
Small is the work that you have done.
You've hit no traitor on the hip?
You've dashed no cup from perjured lip?
You've never turned the wrong to right?
I say you've been a coward in the fight!"

Courage, my friend, and fond greetings—

Bill

Oct. 20, 1880

A voluptuous, large-bosomed middle-aged woman kept her

appointment at two o'clock. Officious in her manner, she sat opposite from me at my desk. Without waiting for a word from me, she cleared her throat and said, "Well, finally there is a woman doctor in this town." "Yes," I agreed.

"I have a house of girls," she announced. "They're all young — no really smart ones. They know only what I have taught them — I want your help. I got money." When I questioned her about the sort of help she expected me to provide, she intimated that she would like the girls to be examined physically once a month. Ten of them. "Can't have them getting sick on me!"

Initially I hesitated, thinking that I was not prepared to make regular visits to a house of prostitution. As a temporary compromise I suggested that I could arrange to see two girls separately at my office at 8 o'clock on Monday mornings. Two months ago I started holding a "questionable" meeting each Monday morning right here. Many developments. I have gotten to know the girls — have discovered that each one has a real affection for their "Madam." Also I have learned that these young women have serious problems. One girl I recognized as having been a pupil in my room at Putnam School when I was a teacher there so many years ago. She had lost weight and had obviously learned the ways of the world and specifically the tricks of after-dark street-walking. She could not look me in the eye.

Another rather pretty girl told me that she was born and raised in the nearby town of Fayetteville, that after both her parents had died leaving her an orphan she was absolutely destitute. Responding to a proposition from a now-married ex-prostitute living nearby, she agreed to go see "kind Madam H. who might find lodging for her in a 'nice house' in the city." She told me that at the time she didn't know what the words "prostitute" "whore" or "pimp" meant.

Ever since my first visit with the Chief of Police concerning the problems of vice and prostitution in the city, I have been appalled at the look-the-other-way and do-nothing policy at the Police Department. Since I am now a board member of the Public

Health Commission, I have already discussed with Dr. M. the condition of health at Madam H.'s home for young girls. Two of the pregnant residents have gonorrhea, another has a full blown case of syphilis. All the others are vulnerable candidates.

During a recent conversation with a friend of mine who is manager at the Wieting Opera House I have learned that I may use an empty basement room once a week. My intention is to invite the girls to meet with me late some afternoon soon, to talk freely about their troubled lives, to ask questions they have never discussed with me at the office, to learn more about themselves, men and babies. I hope I'll be up to answering them.

Dec. 20, 1880

Mrs. D. came into the office obviously distraught. When I questioned her, she denied concern about herself. She was worried about her husband — a Civil War veteran of fifteen years. Says he has a good job, seems to feel well, but at night — many nights — as he lies sleeping beside her, he suddenly trembles, then shakes violently, utters unintelligible sounds — tones of severe fright. Often a muffled scream.

She has never spoken to her husband about these nocturnal thrashings except to ask him in an unconcerned way the following morning if he had had a bad dream. Laughing, he says that he never dreams any more.

"What is it, Doctor?" she asked me. Since the attacks had lately become more frequent and sometimes more severe, she was fearful that he might be on the verge of a mental breakdown.

I questioned her concerning his experiences during the Civil War. She told me that he had dropped out of high school here in order to enlist with an artillery brigade. A group of his pals had decided to sign up together. Fought battles together at Bull Run and Gettysburg. He saw many of his best friends killed. Had often recounted the stories to her with tears in his eyes.

I too feel an uncanny horror even now whenever I listen to

reminiscences about the war. Brother Henry has related fearful tales I shall never forget. He has told me too about his occasional uncontrolable night terrors. I tend to believe that John D. relives the ordeals of over fifteen years ago in his sleep — a form of repetitive nightmare.

My words to Mrs. D. were more conversational than advisory. I told her it might be well now to understand that through the nightmares, her husband was exploding old fears and that by so-doing, he is able to assume his waking, work-a-day life with more equinimity.

Could she understand? Could she manage to soothe him quietly at night when the trembling occurred? Perhaps by the gentle stroking of his back or shoulder and by speaking to him with a quiet, caring, sympathetic tone of voice. I told her that we both — she and I — should be thankful that her husband's waking hours as head of his family were sane and his behavior nonviolent. I assured her that she, with her obvious deep affection for him, could be influential in abating his night-time terrors as well as her own worry.

March 3, 1881

Pa died early this morning in his sleep. Last night he complained that it was hard for him to breathe — thought he must be getting a cold — kept coughing. I put a mustard plaster on his chest, gave him some cough syrup, tucked him into bed with two pillows under his head. He smiled as I blew him a kiss from the doorway. This morning I talked to Pastor C., his good friend. We shall have the funeral here at the house and he will be buried beside Mother in the Manlius cemetery in the spring after the snow has melted. His body will remain in the vault until that time comes. I am sick at heart. Teddy's tears blend with his sobs. I seem unable to comfort him. Fortunately our housekeeper, Mary, and Ted have become good friends. She has promised to stay here during this difficult time and for as long as I need her.

April 15, 1881

Tillie Mae W. arrived at the office on time — not her usual
custom. She had back pains, headaches and her legs, she said,
could barely carry her upstairs at night. Often she was too exhausted to sleep. Six children coming in rapid succession had produced bulging varicose veins — always worse after walking. And
she had a vaginal irritation and discharge. That problem needs
further checking. She was worried about becoming pregnant
again. How was she supposed to protect herself from her demanding husband who often came home drunk? After examining her I
asked her what she had been doing that day. "Recovering," she
said with a deep sigh. She told me that yesterday was "Nail Day."
It was the day she cut all finger and toe nails. Six kids, Bill's and
her own, add up to 160 dirty nails altogether. If she had known
about six kids and their nails before getting married, she swore
she'd still be single.

We talked about schedules — how to cut down on the time she
spent on her feet, about sitting instead of standing to do certain
chores in the kitchen — including ironing the clothes. I realize that
alcohol is becoming a definite and threatening problem to all the
family. Asked if she would bring her husband with her next week
when she returns. I need to talk with them together. I wrote a
note addressed to him, mentioning that I considered it important
to discuss his wife's condition with him. Would he please come
with her at the time of her next appointment?

August 29, 1881

Teddy asked if he might take a cot into the garden to spend the
night. He was fascinated with the fireflies — lured a battery of
them into a wide-mouth canning jar with a perforated lid. It was
late when he finally drifted off to sleep. In the morning when he
came into the house for breakfast — tousled and sleepy-eyed — he
announced in a subdued tone of voice, "Mama, last night I saw

God up in the sky."

I too had seen the northern lights as they played across the late summer sky. The swoop of undulating colors—red, yellow and green—is an unforgettable sight. I told him that in this part of the country if the weather is clear, we can see what the early settlers called the "aurora borealis." And I added, "Teddy, in a way, you are right about seeing God."

Sept. 2, 1881

I spent a long session with Suzy K. today. She is confused now that her baby has been delivered—a sickly specimen of male newborn humanity. Her sixteen years have endowed her with neither love nor wisdom. I remember her well when I was a teacher at Putnam School. At the fifth grade level she ran away from home, apparently having discovered a few predatory boys of the town. She loved the feeling of freedom after the lamp-lighters had made their tour of the darkening streets. At night there was easy money to be gathered in not far from the house where her family lived. No one before had told her how readily the money could be "earned."

But today there were tears. Suzy limped into the office lugging her premature babe. Her blond hair hung in unwashed strands over her shoulders, her face dirt-streaked with tears. She crumpled into the chair by my desk, mewling like a cat. There was no need for her to tell her story.

I called Mary who took her upstairs, peeled off her filthy tattered clothing, bathed both her and the babe. The last I saw her she was curled up on the cot in our back room, with the child now feebly suckling Suzy's little engorged breast.

The problem, of course, involves the future. What is to be done about prostitution and its aftermath in this town? What will happen to Suzy and her unwanted child?

Suzy's predicament obviously now demands justice—justice to Suzy, her child and the community. Without considering what fate she and her child may deserve, I must somehow answer her call for help.

Sept. 5, 1881

The vision of Suzy stays with me — as she looked yesterday when she appeared at my door. And another flash as she appeared dull-eyed in my class at old Putnam School — only a few years ago. She used to sit slumped at her desk fiddling with her pencil or biting her nails. Her body sagged doughy-fat, the expression on her pale face vacant, her nose running. Her blond hair was snarled and unwashed.

Whenever I called on her to recite, she would hang her head and refuse to answer me. She never handed in homework or brought excuses for frequent absences. I never met her parents nor heard from them after Suzy had been given failing grades. I learned later that the change in Suzy had come about during the previous year when her mother had run off with another man. Suzy was left at home more or less in charge of three younger children and, it was reported by neighbors, physically tormented and molested by her father.

Suzy knows nothing about the care of a baby. She has no clothing for the child. Practically no supplies.

I have learned this from her roustabout uncle who came to see me today. The girl and her child are living with him in a one-room shack located on the bank of the canal. He wants to know what to do with her and her "wailing brat."

I wish I knew. I shall call at the house tomorrow.

Next Day

I found the babe unattended — obviously sick. Limp, feverish, diarrhea, breathing irregular, weak cry, eyes rolled back. Suzy was sitting on a step of the back stoop of her brother's shack on the bank of the canal, laughing with a bunch of young men. I took her firmly by the shoulder, told her to clean up the child, wrap him in a blanket.

We were headed for the hospital. She behaved like a puppet. I had Pa's old buggy with Rex tied to the hitching post in front of the shack. We piled in amid stench, tears and cries of dissent as I flicked the whip and shook the reins.

We were off at a fast clip toward the hospital. Dr. W., the best pediatrician in town, happened to be there. He gave the babe a cursory examination and after a brief conversation with Suzy was quick to comprehend the situation. The child must be hospitalized. Suzy should remain—stay close to her baby.

During the night the infant died. The next morning Suzy was again at my door, head hanging low on her chest, eyes downcast, hair degraggled, clothing wrinkled and soiled. Suzy could not ask me for help. She simply stood there—transformed from the fat, unresponsive little girl in my fifth grade class at Putnam School to the thin waif now about to collapse on my doorstep. I called Mary. Arms akimbo, she took one look at Suzy and said, "Doctor, we've got to do something for her."

I lead the way to the dark back room where once before we had cared for her. Mary tucked her into the cot, brought her soup and crackers which she ate hungrily before falling into a deep sleep.

During the next few days Mary taught her to help with some of the simple household tasks about my home and office including the dirty job of cleaning and refilling the oil lamps.

Sept. 7, 1881

I have talked with my old friend, Abby W. who still teaches at Putnam School and who also remembers Suzy. It happens that Abby has been looking for a girl to help her with housework at her big family home where she lives with her mother, an aged invalid. Abby agrees to provide a room for Suzy at the house if she snaps out of her morose moodiness and proves capable of doing the work. After talking with Suzy, I urged Abby to give her a try.

I admit that I still look at Suzy with an uncontrolled feeling of disdain and pessimism. It seems to me that the girl is already one of the many young derelicts among us—foreordained to disaster.

After a month's trial, I met Abby one day at school. She was clearly optimistic. Suzy's appetite was improving. Her ability to pay attention, follow directions and finish simple chores surprised Abby. She has even made friends with Abby's bed-ridden mother who seems to be quite fond of her.

When I stopped in at the W. house some days later, I was gratified to see that Suzy was shiny clean, her blond hair plaited in a neat braid. Showed me her new dress with pride. She told me with a grin that she had learned how to "make a proper bed" and that now she had been carrying food on a tray every day to Mrs. W. in her upstairs room. She likes to talk with her. Told me that doing all these new jobs kept her from "worrying about her dead baby." Still she shows no sign of grief or remorse.

Nov. 2, 1881

Mrs. Libby M. brought her young daughter, aged 13, in to see me today. The office waiting room was full. When their turn came, the girl, Lucy, would not speak or even smile at me. Her complexion was sallow, her eyes downcast, her general attitude withdrawn. The mother complained that her child had "changed —even at home seemed sad, remote, didn't want to go to school, wouldn't even talk to her best chum, refused to answer questions her father and I put to her." After a few moments I told Mrs. M. that if she didn't object I would like to speak with Lucy alone. She was reluctant at first, but finally agreed. Lucy shot me a sharp questioning look.

I put my arm around her and lead her into my small den, asked her to sit beside me on the green settee. She began to cry. I offered her my handkerchief and told her it was perfectly alright to cry. After a pause she mumbled that she was afraid to speak in her mother's presence. When I asked why, she kept her eyes staring at the floor. "I think I am going to die like Aunt Amy. It's because of cancer. . . ." Raising her blouse she said, "You can feel it right here—the lump." Grasping my hand she held it on her small budding breast. Tears again filled her eyes. I told her, no Lucy, this is not cancer, nor anything bad at all. You are becoming a young woman. It is all good and natural. Your other little breast is beginning to grow too and as naturally and beautifully. When we went back into the examining room, Lucy greeted her mother with a broad grin.

The three of us then joined in talking about the mysteries of growing up for both girls and boys. We talked about menstruation and the new sensations which come to a girl at that time. As mother and daughter left the house arm in arm, I felt reassured. I asked Mrs. M. to return next week to discuss the other problem she had on her mind.

November 5, 1881

Teddy came whimpering into my room last night. Earlier I thought I had heard him scream. Sleep-walking, he wandered about the room continuing to cry until I got up, hugged him, spoke gently and after putting cold cloths on his forehead took him into my bed where he finally fell asleep quietly. It took a good half hour before his trembling subsided.

We had been to church that morning—Sunday. The sermon was a long diatribe against Sin. The red-faced minister, with his jowls shaking over his clerical collar, warned his congregation that the Devil was walking among us. He detailed Satan's appearance with explicit words: his skulking body gave out heat, his head encircled with fire, his eyes evil, his horns menacing. In his right hand he brandished a red hot pitchfork and in his other clawed hand he carried a human skull. He brandished a snake-like tail with a sting-pointed tip that flipped about him as he stalked his victims—a child, like Teddy and his Mother, like me. The pastor went on to describe Hell, a fiery place where people

wailed and screeched as flames tortured them. He pounded his
fist on the lectern as with a loud dramatic voice, he warned us
that Hell is a place for Sinners—all Sinners—even children. He
seemed to be finally pointing his long finger at us. I, myself, had
heard enough as I wondered what effect the words would have on
Teddy who sat so solemnly beside me.

When he waked in the morning I asked him about the dream
he had the night before—a bad dream that had made him run to
my bed. He thought for a moment and replied, "Mama, it was
awful. I dreamed the Devil was chasing me. I could feel his hot
fire. I was so scared. He almost caught me. I ran and ran and
tried to call you but the words wouldn't come out!"

It was then that I made up my mind not to take him to that
church again. When I was growing up in the small town of Manlius I believed without question the traditions and moral stan-
dards of behavior I was taught both at home and in the village
church and Sunday School. A human child was born in sin, he
must spend his life earning redemption by thinking so-called pure
thoughts and doing good deeds so that when he died he could
take his place among the angels in Heaven. Somehow though I
always had a hard time imagining myself as an "angel" playing a
harp as I flew among the clouds.

I am today overflowing with questions I hesitate to ask a clergy-
man. Why, for instance, should a child be considered to have
been "born in sin" when a man and a woman have been partners
in creating a new life through an act of love? Love! How does this
relate to the Biblical story of Adam and Eve and their mythical
misbehavior? I am determined to rethink my own ethics of religion and talk often with Teddy about his recurrent worries.

Nov. 15, 1881

Mrs. A. came in to see me as the first patient this afternoon.
Her husband had died last Thursday from cancer. She needed to
talk, wondered how she can manage to cope with life now. His life

insurance she knows will be entirely inadequate. They had practically no savings. Her husband never talked with her about their finances. Probably she can sell the house and with that asset find a smaller place for the three children and herself. She wants to continue sending the children to Putnam School — a wise decision. During the long death wait she has had time to think and in a strange way to grieve. Her friends, so far, are stalwart. I checked her heart and lungs. Basically I did assure her of her own good health and reminded her of the strength she has already demonstrated. She needs encouragement, not medicine.

Before she left she stood silent with eyes cast down, pulled from her pocket a much folded piece of paper and with reticence handed it to me, saying, "Henry left this in a sealed envelope for me to read after the funeral. I don't want to show it to any one else but you."

It was written in her husband's shaky hand.

"When I am gone, and I shall go before you
Think of me not as your disconsolate lover:
Think of the joy it gave me to adore you,
Of sun and stars you helped me to discover.
And this still living part of me will come
To sit beside you in the empty room.
Then all on earth that Death has left behind,
Will be the merry part of me within your mind."

Those two human beings were close in their marraige and growing in their love. Tears were in my eyes too.

November 20, 1881

I have written to the registrar at the Women's Medical College of Pennsylvania in Philadelphia to ask permission for me to spend time there during this Christmas holiday. I would be at the school and hospital as an observer and plan to stay at the home of a friend in Philadelphia.

I have already talked to Billy Stewart's mother who will be "only too glad" to have Teddy stay with them while I am away. Of course Teddy is already looking forward to sharing Bill's room with him.

I have many questions to discuss with the woman doctor in charge of the obstetrical department. And I am curious to inspect the post-partum ward and the nursery. I shall make a special appointment with the director of nurses. Particularly I want to learn how the nurses administer post-partum care to the mothers and how they manage problems for patients following attacks of phlebitis.

I am also interested specifically in diagnosis and management of abnormal fetal position prior to delivery and the presently accepted use of forceps.

                                                    January 6, 1882

Tonight I couldn't sleep. Tried reading the latest Women's Medical Journal, then into the mystery story by my bedside — the print blurred, but my eyelids were not heavy. Happenings of the day replayed themselves in my restive mind. Finally went down to the kitchen, drank a glass of warm milk. I need a friend to talk with me. Desperately I need an understanding friend.

My Journal should not be a one-way source of communication. It isn't. My Best Friend should speak to me! My "Best Friend" could become my other self.

So, quite logically, my Best Friend has obediently written the following words in The Journal:

"Millie . . . You need to be shaken up. Bear in mind that I am not addressing you as if you were Millie, M.D. You are Millie, my best friend. I think you have been hiding behind the M.D. you have worked so hard to add to your name. You have been using your degree as a shield.

First and foremost, Millie, you were a woman, long before you were ever a doctor. You are a strong, feisty woman but a woman afflicted with guilt.

No wonder you are unable to sleep! You have never allowed yourself enough time to complete a full cycle of wakefulness. You have not taken time even to grieve for your parents—neither of them. That grief is bottled up within you. You are deeply troubled without knowing the reason. You have not allowed the tears to flow—ever. Not even in private.

Millie, you don't even take time out anymore to let Teddy know you love him! That young human being, your son, is more sensitive than you realize. He needs a Mother. Give him some of your precious time. Don't take it for granted that he knows you love him. You have been pushing your culpability tight into your being—like a genie. And Millie M.D. is responsible. Tension grows as does your sin of omission, your guilt—the genie. Your guilt finds no safety valve. Your safety valve is to *be* Millie the Woman. Be true to her. Let your tears fall. Laugh when you feel like laughing. Run when you feel like running. Scream when you feel like screaming—somehow—even if it is into your pillow. Love when you feel like loving. Open your heart. Find a living, breathing, flesh and blood friend you can trust. Not just me.

Fling out that bottled up genie. Free yourself, so that as Millie M.D. you can effectively release new talents. Help others to conquer pain and to live more productive lives. You can, you know!

Good night, my Best Friend . . . Sleep peacefully."

July 3, 1882

I delivered a young woman of twenty-five of her first child two months ago. She became progressively more and more depressed, finally being unable to care for herself or the child—let alone her husband who could not explain his wife's hallucinations or mental distress. He had asked Charlotte's mother to come to stay with them until his wife might recover, but she too became unable to cope with the strange situation.

We finally agreed that Charlotte T. must be hospitalized. That afternoon her husband drove her in their buggy to the Institute where she was given a room reserved for use of a staff member — all others filled. Because of her hysterical state Doctor B. gave her a strong sedative. Every hour during the night the nurses checked on her condition. About five o'clock the next morning a nurse discovered that her bed was empty. She had jumped from the unbarred second-floor hospital window to the ground beneath. She was found dead, still clutching a pillow to her breast as if it were a baby.

Mrs. H., the woman's mother, still has two children 12 and 14, at home. She has taken her new grandchild to raise as her own — their own — since both the child's father and Herbert H. have finally agreed to the legal adoption. I shall try to drop in at the house fairly often.

Oct. 25, 1882

Mrs. Polly R. was in the office last week — close to the time for her delivery. All indications pointed toward a normal birthing. Yesterday her labor pains began. Barbara, my new nurse, in her customary efficient way, went to the home late in the afternoon to make preparations for the delivery.

On examination I discovered that unhappily the fetus was now in transverse position — a radical change from last week. Clearly we were faced with a problem. Slowly between pains I managed externally to shift the baby into a cephalic presentation, head firmly in the maternal pelvis. And with Barbara's experienced assistance we maneuvered the safe delivery of a normal female child. No question about it — I had to use forceps. She cried lustily. She was beautiful. Luckily the cord was not at any time compressed or slipped about the child's neck. I am sincerely grateful for the training and understanding of difficult deliveries I gained while studying last year at the Philadelphia Women's Medical College.

Mother and babe are a happy pair today. And so are Nurse

Barbara and I.

January 3, 1883

I knew that Miss Abigail A. had been despondent since her love affair and hope for marriage had suddenly ended before Christmas. However I was not prepared for her sudden appearance here at this house while Teddy was on vacation from school. After talking briefly with her and then listening to a woeful reiteration of her unhappy young life, I suggested that she might stay in one of our rooms upstairs in the "sanitarium" until she was ready again to cope with the changing aspects of her situation. I requested that her sister bring Miss A.'s nightdress and toiletries along with a change of clothing. She tearfully agreed. As she stood, she clutched at her abdomen as if in severe pain. I put my arm about her waist helping her to ascend the steep stairway. Suddenly I realized that she was in frightful pain. Screaming, she was about to collapse.

I called Ted who was amazed to see the spectacle of silver globules of mercury bouncing down the wooden stairs. Miss A. had swallowed quicksilver in an attempt to end her life. Suicide was thwarted as the heavy balls of mercury passed rapidly and safely through her alimentary canal, being expelled rectally.

Armed with a glass jar, Teddy caught the run-away tiny balls of mercury as they escaped her tortured body from beneath her rumpled skirts. Teddy appeared to be fascinated with his new role and I know he will never forget the experience.

Within a week, Abigail, with the affection, good food and attention she received here, seemed to recover her mental and physical equilibrium. She has gone to her sister's home to stay for a few weeks and will report to me twice a week until I am convinced that she is well on the way to complete recovery — as complete as possible at this stage of her life. I shall follow her progress closely.

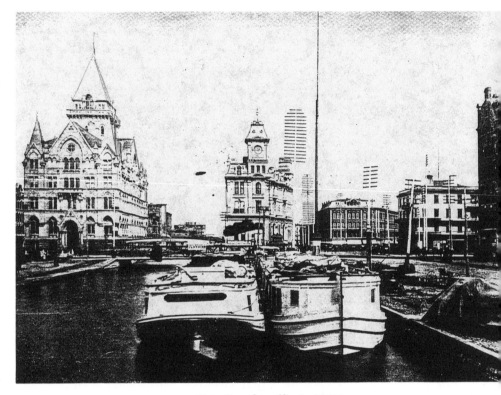

Erie Canal traffic in 1883.
(Courtesy of The Erie Canal Museum)

June 18, 1883

Teddy and I boarded the canal packet boat early Saturday morning, headed for Rome where I planned to visit a former patient who was suffering through the last stages of breast cancer. She had written asking if I would please visit her. The day was warm and sunny. Teddy was in fine spirits—whistling "Low Bridge, Everybody Down" as we crossed over the gangplank near the downtown weighlock building.

We found seats atop the old barge so that we could see what

was going on at both sides of the canal as we edged along at less than five miles an hour. The ancient mule that was towing the barge seemed weary and at times almost in pain. I suppose mules can have rheumatism too.

As we drifted along at the mule's worse than slow pace the teacher-in-me came to the surface as I began to regale Ted with some of the more pertinent facts about the canal. About how, in 1817, Rome—our destination—was the starting place of the canal where the first shovelful of dirt was dug; about how 300 bridges were built along the 363 miles of canal—now connecting Buffalo and Albany—Lake Erie and the Hudson River.

In New York State before the winter freezes us over, I told him of how people and goods of all sorts can be transported from as far west as Chicago through the Great Lakes along the Canal and down the Hudson River from Albany to New York City harbor.

"Dewitt Clinton's Ditch" now has 83 locks to make it possible for a barge to be lifted up the long rise from the Hudson River to the level of Lake Erie. The early laborers, many of whom had come as immigrants from Ireland and Germany, worked long hours with picks and shovels. Scores of workers died of malaria and other diseases during the many hot months of construction. Everyone then thought that malaria came from the vapors rising from the swamps in these parts. Those men who survived settled in the towns and cities along the course of the canal. In fact much of our present population along its route are children and grand-children of those early workmen.

It was for Ted a first-time experience. At the start of our trip, as we approached the Lodi Street lock, he was able to learn how the lockmaster controls the inflow and outflow of water to allow the passage of one barge after the other. First toward the west and then toward the east.

At one of the towns I encouraged Teddy to debark and run alongside the boat on the towpath to talk to the "canawlers," maybe to have a chance to hold the reins of the slow-moving old mule.

Below decks with the other passengers we were served luncheon on collapsible tables—a delicious meal of beef stew, potato salad, corn and beans with cider or tea and chocolate cake for dessert. On the houseboats we passed we saw women peeling potatoes, sewing, washing their hair on board or dunking their dirty babies into tubs of water. Small boys fished from the deck or dove from the shore to swim in the canal. Men worked the farms along the way. As we passed small towns we could see the activity within the shops and stores lining the canal.

Small groups of men and women were buying or selling. Some old men sat in front of the stores—watching the barges as they passed, their chairs tilted against the buildings—whittling pieces of wood, smoking or chewing tobacco and spitting with a wide arc into a convenient cuspidor. At Oneida more passengers boarded the packet.

Soon Teddy found a friend of his own age. They came to me surprised to discover that there were berths below deck where people could sleep at night—the men's section divided from the women's by a thick curtain.

Leaving the packet boat at Rome, we boarded a horse-car to take us to the street where Mrs. S. now lives. My former patient, obviously pleased to see us, had many questions for me. She had invited her grandson to rollerskate with Ted, so we were assured of privacy in our conversation over a cup of tea. Ella S. seemed chiefly concerned about how much longer she has to live. Of course I don't know, but we did philosophize a bit about the need to live each day to its utmost. In appearance, she is pale and cadaverously thin but her voice was strong and her face lit up as she spoke. Obviously she is receiving adequate care at home. I spoke with the nurse who is staying with her.

When it came time for us to go, I felt the friendly squeeze of a hand and watched the tear in her eye spill down her cheek as we said goodbye.

At five o'clock Teddy and I were on the New York Central train chugging back to Syracuse. The sound of the engine's toot, the puff of steam, the sense of the engine's power, the conductor's whistle and his cadenced call of "Al-l-l Aboard" filled me with nostalgia. I remembered a long-ago train ride with Edward—a honeymoon. Teddy sat quietly beside me on the window side watching the landscape pass by.

As we finally rolled slowly into the center of the city of Syracuse, he seemed fascinated with the sight of women who leaned out of second story windows of the houses bordering the tracks: men staggerd drunk—in and out through the swinging slatted doors of saloons—dogs barked as young children stopped in their play to gape at the slow-moving train on its noisy chug to the station through the center of the city.

July 1, 1883

It was not until I had been a practicing physician for five years that I was admitted as a member of the Commission for the Syracuse Department of Public Health. The spread of tuberculosis has been like wild fire in the city and outlying areas. There have been recent outbreaks of typhoid fever, typhyus, cholera, measles, scarlet fever, whooping cough, diphtheria and small pox, making it necessary to quarantine many of the houses where such patients were known to be living. Health of the school children of the city has been the chief concern. Both Departments of Education and Public Health joined in attempting to control the rampant spread of communicable diseases. Official notices of quanantine in the form of warning placards have been posted at the front doors of all designated houses. No visitors or unauthorized persons are allowed to enter. Children known to have been ill or exposed to these diseases are not allowed to return to school until a public health official grants permission or lifts the quarantine.

Not only am I involved through active membership on the Board of Health, but also from time to time I take my turn as school physician. All children prior to being admitted to public school must be vaccinated against smallpox.

June 8, 1884

The funeral of my old Manlius friend, Minnie Edwards, lasted too long. The house held a heavy fragrance of fading roses. The entire house was dark; doors and windows closed, all draperies drawn. As I sat in a straight uncomfortable chair near the open casket, I could feel myself growing faint in spite of myself. The pale shrouded remains of 60-year-old Minnie — still wearing steel-rimmed glasses — had breathed her last painful breath. Old Pastor Adams' lugubrious voice droned on and on in a monotone accompanied by sniffs and sobs from female mourners as my heavy head sank jerkily onto my chest.

The immediate family were seated in the upstairs hall. I could hear childish whisperings and an occasional uncontrolled gasp or giggle. Someone played "Rock of Ages" on the piano and we all stood and sang — some louder than others.

Carriages were lined up along the street in front of the house. Now and then I could hear a whinney from a restless horse. At last it was time to drive to the cemetery. I rode with Professor D. and his wife. As we arrived at the entrance gate the heavens opened up pouring down a warm spring rain in sheets. The freshly dug grave looked to me like a gateway to the River Styx as the rivulets streamed from a pile of earth into the open pit.

Eight bearers carried the casket to the brink of the grave. Slowly the apparatus, already in place, lowered the wet flower-covered coffin into its crypt.

We all stood solemnly soaked, circling the grave as Pastor Adams repeated the familiar words, "From dust thou art to dust returneth . . ." I was able to think in terms of Mud — not "dust." As I glanced away from the grave toward the granite tombstones surrounding us, suddenly to my mind the obelisks became phallic symbols.

Subsequently I became conscious that a tall, sandy-haired gentleman was holding a large black umbrella over my head. I looked up at him, nodded a thank-you.

As the knot of sad friends dispersed he walked by my side still holding the protective but dripping umbrella. He introduced himself—Andrew DeMott—a friend of the dead woman's husband. When he graciously offered to drive me home in his carriage, I accepted. We were both soaked from the torrential rain.

At my door I invited him to come for tea next Sunday afternoon.

Mr. Andrew DeMott did come for tea the following Sunday. About five o'clock Teddy returned from a fishing expedition with Bill. Ruddy-faced and grinning he showed us his bountiful whitefish catch, shook hands with Mr. DeMott and disappeared. Conversation with Mr. D. had few lapses. I would like to know him, to count him as a friend.

January 5, 1885

My concern last evening centered about the impression I would make on Andrew's friends—I, a woman doctor. Strange to feel so self-conscious. The occasion I refer to was an anniversary party at the Nick Peters' home. Andrew wanted me to meet some of his friends.

I wore my new dress to the dinner party. Emily Johnson had designed it from the blue silk material I had purchased on sale at Lacy's Store last fall. It is beautiful. I have had no occasion until now to wear such raiment. It has small self-covered buttons decorating the bodice with modified leg-o-mutton sleeves and a long full skirt.

As I combed my hair I spent much more time than I usually do. This amounts to a confession to myself. With a hand mirror I inspected my left profile as it was reflected from the looking glass over my dresser. I noticed that I had pulled my somewhat curling hair straight back over my ear to the coil on top of my head. Turning, I compared my right profile to the left. Right is more

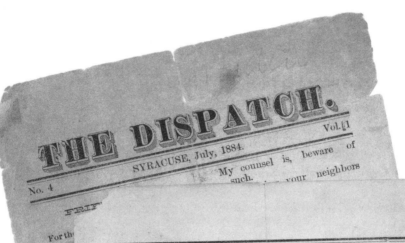

THE DISPATCH.

Vol. 1

SYRACUSE, July, 1884.

No. 4

My counsel is, beware of such. . . . . your neighbors

FRI. . .

For th. . .

H. . .

DISPATCH.

PUBLISHED MONTHLY

W. H. STEWART, } EDITOR & PUBLISHER.

E. H. DANN, *Associate.*

TERMS:

Single Copies, — — — — —	$.01
Six Months - - - - - - - - - -	$ .06
1 year, — — — — — —	$.10

By mail, 10 cents extra.

All communications should be addressed to,—

THE DISPATCH,
57 E. Jefferson, St.,
Syracuse, N. Y.

☞ We will exchange with all amateur papers.

ADVERTISING RATES given on application at this office.

OUR NEXT NUMBER.

As most of our readers are going to summer resorts to spend the season, and as we have always gone away ourselves, we have concluded we will continue doing the same.

But the question is, what will we do about the August number of our paper.

But as we hope to be back by the first of September, we have decided, if our subscribers do not object, to print an eight paged sheet which will take the place of our August and September numbers.

Will deliver it about the middle of the month.

Amateur News.

N. A. P. A.

For President,
Ralph Metcalf.

For Vice-president,
Geo. J. Boehm.

Chautauqua for the N. A. P. A. convention in '85.

Syracuse for the Esapa convention in '85.

Mail by the Salt City Bundle, sent by Messrs. Cherry and Smith.
Papers mailed the 7th of each month

Who says the "Gauntlet" is a campaign paper?

Tattered copy of the Dispatch, *1884.*

interesting—nose more patrician. I never noticed the difference before.

I then studied the view of my head from the rear—the small coil of hair wound from the nape of my neck to the top of my head seemed all right, especially with the tortoiseshell comb tucked in just beneath it. A touch of elegance, I thought to myself.

The shock came when I turned to take a careful frontal look at my face with the thought that I should attempt to see myself as Andrew sees me. The two lateral halves of my face are not identical! I covered the right side of my face with my hand. That left half somehow looked familiar to me—stern, business-like, serious. My chin seemed to have a tendency to jut out and my lips from that side formed a severe straight line. There are fine wrinkles at the far corner of my left eye. And for the first time I noticed scattered gray hairs at the temple. Not many.

Then I covered the left side of my face and was surprised to see a different me. My mouth had a half smile, the nostril less flared. And my right eye looked back at me as if it were about to wink—almost mischievously.

The entire right side of my face, especially as I loosened the tightly pulled hair over my ear, revealed an unfamiliar feminine reflection. For a change I'll present the "right" side of myself the next time I am photographed!

By the time we arrived in his carriage at the Peters' home I felt quite comfortable at Andrew's side. He even complimented me. And as the evening came to a close and we were driving home, Andrew kissed me.

February 25, 1885

The extent of prostitution in our city is not generally known. Physicians do recognize the spread of veneral disease and are cognizant of the increased number of babies born with physical defects. Blindness, mental retardation, other physical abnormalities are the signs. But what about the influence on the victims' parents, the grandparents and other relatives of the infected children? The roots of many old and respected families in this city seem tangled with disease and rot.

Poverty too exists in this town—as does hunger and crime. These conditions, seldom publicized, meld into producing problems which, it seems to me, we must all face and help to obliterate.

The other day I copied this bit of pertinent verse from a book of poetry. The words seem appropos to my thoughts today.

THE OUTCAST
(Author unknown)

"Shunned of women and scorned by men
Brazen and bold along the streets
Courting the stares of all she meets,
Flaunting her shame where'er she can,
A mocking laugh, a mirthless smile—
Not one home to take her in.

Here walks the Outcast, daughter of sin.
Pure hopes once dwelt in a future bright—
Her life to be filled with love and light.
We eye her with misery, laugh her to scorn,
Watch her with malice, disdain and a frown
As she curses her God and the day she was born.

Remember the merciless world she meets,
How deep she sinks in the mire of streets!
Can we pray with sincerity for such as she,
Refusing to help—simply let her be!

Remember how Jesus, the Lord, was seen
To pity and pardon the Magdalene."

It was snowing as I walked home from my downtown office in the Hendricks Block tonight. I was shivering and still so cold that after a cup of tea and a sandwich I headed upstairs for a hot bath.

I find after a long busy day that soaking in the warm water of the bathtub can provide effective therapy for me. In addition to being comforting to weary bones, I can use the steamy silence to help resolve some of the nagging questions that sometimes prod my confused mind for hours after I have returned home.

I have been giving thought to the growing existence of prostitution in this city. I realize that the problems of womankind have been a societal concern for centuries. One aspect of that concern comes sharply into my consciousness. Significantly Men, representing Church and State, have been our judges, the "morality" assessers, the law-makers and have been the so-called benefactors of their communities over the years.

From the biblical story of Adam and Eve, we have read that it was Eve who eventually became the temptress with apple in hand. Sex became identified with "original sin." And now in the nineteenth century during a time when rights for women are being publicly sought as equal to those of men, we as women must ask thought-provoking and intelligent questions.

Why should the prostitute be the culprit punished?

What of the pimp who procured her? It is he who gains financially from her illegal, tutored, provocative activity. What of the continued police protection of the madam in her bawdy House of Prostitution?

What of the men who leave their marriage beds and disregard vows in order to satisfy lust?

What of the young girls and children who are sold into "white slavery," who are transported across state and national borders to be lost forever?

What of the corruptible police protection provided our well-known barrooms and second-floor dance-halls? The very Civic Policemen supported through our people's taxes become the generators of vice! What of their protecting the pimps and madames for on-going fees? What about their nonchalant supervision of our entire "red light districts"?

Whose responsibility is it to care for the illegitimate and unwanted babies of this growing community? Why?

Who takes notice of the spread of venereal disease? Is the
spread controllable?

What about the unemployment of the once pert and pretty
lasses now grown fat, flatulent and untrained except for their
talented sexual antics? What of the wives innocently infected by
their own mates?

What about the breakdown of families? The children.

What about the early initiation of young college men into the
brothels of this town — the pleasant lure and snare of alcohol?

What about the role of the Church in dealing with unsavory
social problems?

What about the education of our young at home and in our
schools?

These questions confounded me as I soaked.

April 2, 1885

This morning Doctor B. stopped me as I was leaving the hospital. Asked if I would be willing to serve on the Medical College
Admissions Committee of which he is chairman. He explained
that the task would involve interviewing candidates during the
spring and summer — especially the female applicants. Although I
was on my way to the office and a bit breathless, I told him I
would probably give him an affirmative answer.

I have written him a letter letting him know that I consider it
an honor to be asked to serve on his committee. I look forward to
meeting the first candidate — be it he or she - male or female — in
the College admissions office. I told him that I shall look forward
as well to discussing other aspects of the responsibility with him
and members of his committee. I am especially interested in en-
couraging more women to study medicine.

Already I wondered what their answers would be to the inevitable questions: "What makes you want to become a doctor?" "Do

you now or in the future plan to be married?" "How do you feel about having children?" "Are you prepared for the long grind?"

I am ready and eager to discuss these matters and many more with any young men or women who wish to apply at our Medical College.

September 16, 1885

I have had interesting and revealing conversations with both the men and women medical school candidates. All the women I spoke with expressed confidence that their approach to caring for patients would differ from male doctors they have known. I interpreted their approach as being far from scientific. More nurturing in essence. However, responses spread over a wide spectrum, depending on background—family, life/death concerns and actual experience. One young woman told me that her father is a country practioner, that from the time she was a child she has made house calls with him, has helped him in his office. Furthermore her only brother who—in the family's expectation—was studying to become a physician at Columbia, had died last winter from an attack of pneumonia. Now she is convinced that studying medicine is up to her!

Few women had any conception of what effect sexual denigration can have on self-respect nor do they understand the reality of competition with men in this profession. Only one woman looked like a fighter to me—she plans to go to Africa as a medical missionary!

Many of the men were frank in admitting that they wished to become influential in their communities, to be respected and to be able to make money, "To do good in the world." On the other hand there were some young men whose friends or family members had known death. Were those deaths preventable? Their concerns were real. One man spoke about the vulnerability of the human species. He had visions of working in a laboratory—wanted to be another Louis Pasteur or Robert Koch.

Few candidates—men or women—were properly prepared academically nor did one of them evidence willingness, by further study, to improve chances for acceptance. None of them seemed to me to understand the extent of dedication required of time, of energy, of money, of self.

Personally, I was surprised to realize that at least in my estimation, only five or six men or women I have so far interviewed, would be viable candidates to be accepted in this Medical School.

September 20, 1885

The coming to Syracuse of a famous Minstrel Show had been advertised for weeks. I have been having my nose to the grindstone for months, so that when Andrew asked me to attend the production at the Wieting Opera House last Saturday evening I was eager in voicing my enthusiasm. This was another first experience for me. I didn't know what to expect. I had a preconceived notion that all the performers would be negro.

As the curtain went up the impression I had was that every singer on the platform had black skin, except for the two white end-men. I quickly realized that all the men were white—that their faces had been blackened and made up. They all wore black curly wigs and white gloves. Spoke with the unmistakable southern drawl.

I was delighted as they sang the familiar songs from the south —from before and after the Civil War. Some of them danced with their soft shoes and natural rhythm from one end of the stage to the other. They told jokes as the interlocutor shot questions to the end-men who vied with each other in making the audience laugh.

At times I found myself not laughing at the jokes. I was distracted by a familiar bald-headed man seated directly in front of me. A balding surgeon I knew well. I would recognize his face anywhere, but I had never before viewed his head from the rear.

When he laughed, he laughed heartily. Even the skin of his

pink bald head wrinkled — wrinkled into an extended back-of-his-head smile.

Andrew hadn't noticed.

Afterward my new friend Andrew drove me home. We had hot tea and crumpets in front of a blazing fire in the grate.

Dec. 20, 1885

Andrew had asked me to go with him to attend a twenty-fifth wedding anniversary party at his friend's home. Nick Peters likes to fish — has a lodge somewhere in the Adirondack Mountains where the two of them often go. Nick's friends are Andrew's friends. At the party — much interesting talk and good-natured laughter. No separating the men from the women as so often happens at a dinner party. The midnight buffet was delicious. Poached salmon.

And later Andrew kissed me good night.

February 13, 1886

My informal lectures at the Syracuse W.C.A. (Women's Christian Association)* are taking on a new momentum. A young woman has been hired to look after small children who have been showing up with their mothers. Occasional childish outbursts have been happily eliminated now that they can be cared for in another room. We have been discussing domestic problems — from how to deal with bored husbands to the growing need of

* The organization preceding our YWCA was called simply "WCA." Beginning simply in Syracuse, its primary purpose was "to care for homeless working girls." The first boarding home was established in 1886, the residents being admitted only "after rigorous and thorough examination." The first applicant was "a young lady student from the Medical School."

The WCA's secondary purpose was to save young women from "falling into sin," to advocate, to promote enriching experiences, to oversee proper employment, to broaden interest among Syracuse women — an important factor in expanding WCA work.

understanding rebellious sons and daughters.

Last week I passed out pencils and slips of paper asking the fifteen or twenty in the room to list subject matter they would like to have me talk about. Topics ranged from—what should I keep on hand in our medicine cabinets and why, to how do I know when I am going through the change of life, to what can I do for colds and sore throats, to what are we supposed to tell our daughters these days about menstruation, to myths about certain old wives' tales and the use of specific patent medicines and herbs, to what causes food poisoning and on and on—to the causes of miscarriage and rights for women.

I like to stress over and over again the importance of good posture, walking for exercise, regular airing out of our homes, the need for all of us to eat more vegetables and fruits. *No* alcohol or guns in our homes.

I also put emphasis on the need to guide the choice of books our children read, the importance of making frequent visits to our children's classrooms and of having frank discussions with their teachers.

I like to remind the mothers that only a few years ago the Syracuse Board of Education received national recognition for excellence of our teaching methods and for our sustained academic achievement among the boys and girls attending our growing number of public schools. The last census revealed substantial increase in the number of school-age children in this community.

I am impressed with the ladies' enthusiastic interest in joining freely into the discussions. I shall be widening my own sphere of reading and knowledge. . . . I must.

March 14, 1886

A new patient, Mary Ann C., looked skeptically at me, raising one thick black eyebrow and tapping her right foot nervously. I noticed that her fingernails had been bitten to the quick. Her face was flushed and she persisted in shrugging her shoulders.

Obviously she was worried . . . spoke of gas pain, "headaches." We talked about self-respect. It is important to honor every organ in our bodies, to be alert to the messages they send—each one. Our brain is the guardian of our bodies—our whole selves.

I knew from what she had told me that she has been really sick. I said, "I know you do want to get better. I know that you are concerned about your health. Otherwise, you wouldn't have come to see me." She nodded. I proceeded to tell her that I was completely unable to help her unless she helped herself. (My old saw!) I asked her if she thought medicine I might give her would contain some specific magic. Again she nodded. Again I explained that medicine might help her but only if she allowed it to do so. If medicine desensitizes an isolated pain, it may affect the whole patient. She continued to glare at me now with both eyebrows raised and a scowl wrinkling her forehead.

I told her that I was going to ask her a series of questions, that I wanted her to answer them as honestly as she could.

I told her again to realize that I had known her for only a short time, that my knowledge of her problems was necessarily slight. I asked her to relax. To try to be as forthright with me as I was with her.

I told her that as I examined her we could talk. Her answers to me about herself, the life she lived, her habits were just as important to me as if she had an elevated temperature or that she had a pain in her abdomen. She smiled with a glimmer of understanding.

I asked her when last she had walked a mile rather than taking the trolley letting the horse do the work. I asked her about the sweets she had devoured between meals, about what she had eaten for breakfast, about when she had last weeded her garden with the sun shining warmly on her back. I asked her pointed questions about how she felt toward her husband and toward each one of their four growing children, about her friends. Suddenly tears began streaming down her cheeks as she sat at the end of the examining table, her head bowed onto her chest. Her body convulsed with sobs. She confessed she felt miserable, that her marriage was unhappy, that she feared the future.

As she gradually recovered her equinimity, I told her about a class I was giving in a small room at the WCA. I thought she might be interested in joining the group. I would personally welcome her if she could come Tuesday morning at ten o'clock.

There would be a few young women coming together whom I thought she would like to meet. I explained that my informal talks once a week concern the oft-times hidden inner strengths we are all endowed with, capable of leading each of us into living more healthy more productive lives. She seemed pleased to be asked to join the class.

I gave her no medication. Asked her to return in two weeks.

May 7, 1886

Mrs. Marian P., mother of four children aged 2, 5, 6 and 8, moved slowly from her chair in the waiting room to my private office. Her husband had died last week as a result of injuries suffered from an accident at the factory where he worked. She knew she was pregnant again, now complaining of sustained weariness, headaches, pain in her legs from pressure on varicose veins, greater tenderness in her breasts than she remembered from previous pregnancies. This being her first prenatal visit she told me that she believed she was no more than five months along in spite of her appearance. We discussed a method of determining an expected date of delivery by adding seven days to the date of her last menstrual period and counting ahead ten lunar months.

On examination I heard two separate foetal heartbeats. No doubt. In spite of her normal physical development, her abdomen was enlarged beyond expectation for a five-month pregnancy. As I shared my finding with her she stared glassy-eyed at me before bursting into tears. How was she ever to manage six children alone!

I comforted her as best I could and asked her to return to see me in two weeks—sooner if her symptoms did not improve. I stressed the need to keep her legs elevated as much as she could and to avoid drinking coffee or consuming food which obviously disagreed with her. Most of all she needs help. We talked about the need to keep her family together and discussed practical methods of finding some household help. She has no family living here.

June 16, 1886

Teddy graduated as Salutatorian from High School last evening—second highest academically in his class. Much to my surprise. The exercises were held in the Wieting Opera House just as mine from Medical School were eight years ago. No Grandmother, no Grandfather and no Father to witness the occasion. How proud they all would have been of him—especially when he stood up to speak before his classmates and their gathered relatives and friends. He knew them all, it seemed to me.

After a coached dramatic pause he smiled quietly at the audience and with no notes, recited his senior speech, an essay titled "The Mind Cure." I wonder what inspired him. The heart of his message was suggested probably from what he has seen happen to patients at my office and sanitarium. And besides he has been doing a great deal of reading at the public library. He has seen ladies come to confer with me about their various ills and complaints. He knows that many of them have changed their habits of poor nutrition, lack of exercise and doomed attitudes toward domestic problems. He has listened to me harp about spending more hours out-of-doors, about finding wholesome use of leisure time, about using hands and minds creatively.

He knows I don't know much about cooking, but he has heard me talk about what makes up a nutritious meal. He has probably chuckled often when he has heard me advising a woman how to dress more comfortably, about ways to stop an argument, about finding new ways to enjoy life within the family.

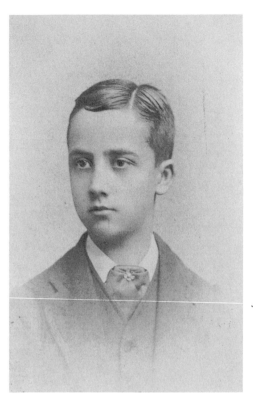

Ted's graduation from high school, June 1886.

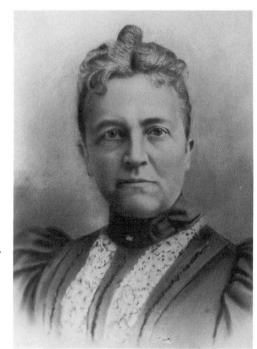

Millie at the age of 40.

In the meantime he has learned about Hippocrates and why he is known even now as the Father of Medicine. It came as no surprise to him that the Greek, Hippocrates, believed that Man brings disease on himself by disobeying the rules of Nature, that if a man has faith in his physician and in himself by respecting Nature, disease can be cured or at least slowed in its ravages. An individual has the power to correct a disordered function of his body by increased control of his thinking processes. Therefore, he concluded, the human mind can positively influence the cure of disease.

He spoke well, but I think he will never want to study medicine. He says that his plan will be to begin freshman courses at the University in the fall with the aim of becoming a newpaper writer. He now has a summer job working at the *Syracuse Daily Standard*, as a cub reporter.

After the commencement exercises were concluded there was a general intermingling of families and friends in the mood of excited celebration and congratulation to all members of the class. I was not surprised that Teddy arrived home well after midnight. He came into my room and gave me a warm, quiet hug in the dark.

August 16, 1886

Ethel T., a 37-year-old woman who came to see me for the first time today, referred by one of her quilt-making friends, complained that she had been spotting blood between menstrual periods, had pain on intercourse, no appetite. She explained that she had been unable to recover from grief and depression since the loss of both her parents from heart ailments and a ten-year-old son from drowning. Three losses within the year.

Physical examination revealed enlargement of the uterus with some bleeding and tenderness. I arranged for her to see Dr. B whose diagnostic and surgical ability I have long respected. After attempting to allay her fears, I promised to see her daily if and when hospitalization occurs. I am sure she is suffering from cancer.

August 20, 1886

Annie McM., my patient for many years, had sent her husband to the office to tell me of his wife's discomfort. She had been suffering from intermittent pain for the past week and felt unable to exert strength sufficient to make an office visit. I arranged to make a house call late in the afternoon. He was obviously worried.

She complained of severe pain in the area of her right shoulder in spite of no recent muscular strain. There was mild tenderness in the right lower quadrant of her abdomen—no rigidity. An enema had not relieved the discomfort. She had no appetite, looked worried, pale. Pulse rapid. Last menstrual period ten weeks ago. While preparing breakfast for her husband and three children that morning, she had suddenly "felt faint." Went back to bed where she had stayed all day.

After brief discussion with her husband I recommended immediate hospitalization and consultation with Dr. B. I feared internal bleeding from the rupture of a tubal pregnancy. Surgery performed that evening verified my diagnosis. I shall plan to see her as often as I can while she is a patient at the Good Shepherd Hospital. Dr. B. is confident that she will make a complete recovery and be able to have more children if the couple so desire.

August 25, 1886

With increased frequency I need to refer certain patients to Dr. B. and Dr. Y. for them to assess surgical problems. I note with some satisfaction that they seem to respect my judgment in making preliminary diagnoses.

Consistently I am refused operating privileges. I really don't want them anyway now. However, the surgeons often assign post-

operative care to me and call me in for staff rounds for the gyne-
cological and obstetrical patients. Often a few medical students
are invited to join us.

The Director of Nurses, Miss MacD., has requested conferences
with me in her hospital office to discuss possible changes in the
nursing care of difficult patients. I appreciate her confidence in
my judgment. Our mutual respect is developing into friendship.

August 29, 1886

I have presumed for some time that Andrew and I would eventually be married. We are both devoted to the idea of marriage to
each other and to the life together we are hoping to establish. The
date has been set for September twenty-ninth. I have mailed the
hand-written invitations.

We have asked Dr. Wellesley P. Coddington to officiate. We
intend to invite only a few of our friends and most congenial
relatives to join us at this house for the ceremony and reception.
Mary and Minnie are eager to take over the kitchen preparations
and since flowers are few in the garden, I have asked my friend
Fred at the Flower Mart to provide a few appropriate potted
palms. He assured me that there will be a fine centerpiece for the
table and flowers for the mantel. Already my good neighbors
have offered to provide dainty sandwiches, fruitcake and chocolate delicacies as well. And there will be punch served from
Mother's beautiful hand-painted bowl.

In addition we shall have champagne! This wedding of ours will
be a gala occasion — a small gala occasion.

September 10, 1886

Ted has begun classes as a freshman at Syracuse University, but
will continue to live at home at least for awhile. Home, with my
secondary office as part of it, will continue to be located right
here on East Fayette Street where many of my patients are used to

finding me. Besides from here it is but a short walk to Andrew's office.

Andrew seems pleased that my professional interests will continue unabated. He says with a twinkle in his eye, "Millie, you keep on tending your ailing women and I shall keep on tending my metals."

We both look forward to the time when we shall perhaps be able to travel without the responsibilities which keep us both anchored here. How I revel at the thought of being able to journey around the world with Andrew! I wonder if it will ever happen. Of course, I do not intend to retire from my profession for many years to come.

Sept. 11, 1886

Mrs. Etta T. came into my office yesterday with her nine-year-old Mary who was crying and holding her right hand over her ear. The pain had been keeping the child and her mother too, awake for three nights. The ear drum was red and distended; tenderness over the mastoid area. I sent them directly to see Doctor A. who diagnosed the problem as being a severe infection which had extended to the mastoid bone. He operated on the child this morning, after having had an altercation with the mother who had tried to force her way into the operating room. Since I happened to be in the hospital at the same time, I was able to divert the mother's attention, assuring her of the capability of Dr. A. to perform the surgery. Later I helped to wheel the child back to her room. When she had regained consciousness with effects of the aenesthetic wearing off, Dr. A. came into the room. We were both relieved to see the girl's first smile — no paralysis of the facial nerve. I have seen too often a resulting permanent one-sided facial paralysis.

October 13, 1886

Our wedding day developed into a beautiful fall afternoon. Colors of the leaves and fall flowers spectacular. I shall never forget the beauty of that afternoon.

I do admire and love Andrew, although it occurs to me that I have not yet told him so. I daresay however, that he is a staunch believer in my silent devotion — as I am in his.

Andrew's parents came to our wedding from Oswego. They had only recently celebrated their own Golden Wedding anniversary. The Chancellor of the University attended with his wife, as well as members of the medical faculty and their spouses. Nick Peters and his wife too. Of course Teddy and his friends — a few. And Uncle William came from New Haven with his wife. It has been years since last I saw them.

I wore a handsome new dress fashioned from ecru lace with a high collar and a floor sweeping skirt. No veil. And I carried one red rose. Andrew wore his best gray suit with a rose in his lapel. We had no attendants — no music except the lovely sound of our friends' voices and Lohengrin's Wedding March played on our piano by our good nieghbor's daughter, ten-year-old Constance, as the time came for us to walk toward Dr. Coddington who was standing in front of the fireplace with its flower bedecked mantel. The ceremony was simple and promptly concluded. Sociability with our friends was delightful. Ted never stopped smiling.

My travel outfit was a new seal-brown suit made of a smooth worsted material. Luxurious. And a feathered hat to match in color. We boarded the 7:40 p.m. train for Chicago planning on the way west to visit Andrew's friends in Milwaulkee and Minneapolis. The tour of Yellowstone Park as passengers in an orange-colored coach drawn by four black houses was spectacular — especially the sight of Old Faithful spouting its high flourish of water every hour of the day and night. We were also amazed at the number of free roaming wild animals throughout the Park. It was a beautiful trip.

On our return Ted showed us a notice he had clipped from the *Syracuse Standard* of September 30. It read:

> "Dr. Amelia Dann DeMott, whose marriage took place yes-
> terday at her home to Mr. Andrew J. DeMott, is expected to
> return on November 1 to reopen her main office in the Hend-
> ricks Block. Dr. DeMott graduated with the class of 1878 from
> Syracuse Medical College and has studied obstetrics and gyne-
> cology at the Woman's Medical Colleges in both New York City
> and Philadelphia.
>
> "Mr. DeMott, formerly a resident of Oswego, is owner and
> manager of the Empire Metal Co., a firm manufacturing metal
> alloys on East Water Street of this city.
>
> "Mr. and Mrs. DeMott will be occupying Mrs. Dann's former
> residence on East Fayette Street upon their return to this city."

January 13, 1887

Very early Monday morning as I was walking along Bank Alley on the way to the Pharmacy in order to refurbish my office medical supplies. I slipped on a patch of ice. I crumpled to the walk-way. My right arm as I attempted to break the fall took the impact of the icy slide. Luckily I didn't hit my head! Hat, medical bag and purse went flying. Not a soul was around at that early hour except one young man who suddenly appeared at the corner, spotted my predicament and on the run, came to my rescue. I knew there had been a fracture. Numbness prior to excruciating pain, sudden swelling.

After retrieving my possessions, my rescuer insisted on accompanying me to the hospital in his rig which he had left down the street with his horse reined and secured to a hitching post in front of the Pharmacy. I knew that once I could be helped into the hospital I would find a friend to care for me and my broken bone.

Young Doctor John A., on duty at the time, gave me a shot of morphine, set the fractured radius, applied the plaster cast and arranged for me to occupy a hospital bed for the rest of the day.

A young nurse in senior cap and uniform, pushed me in a wheel-chair to a private room.

As the nurse helped me onto the bed, our eyes locked. Suddenly I recognized her. She was none other than Suzy K. — tall, slim, calm and smiling. Morphine was beginning to affect me: vision somewhat blurred. Still my distorted recognition of Suzy at that moment astonished me. She arranged pillows to make me comfortable and to support my arm. I could almost feel her compassion as she stroked the wet plaster of the cast and spoke kind words of concern for me. She quickly assured me that she would notify my husband at his office, explaining to him about the accident and requesting him to call for me at the Good Shepherd Hospital later in the day. She then asked permission to stay with me — eager to talk for a few moments.

The saga of Suzy fascinates me. After two years of living with Miss Abby and caring for her dying mother, Suzy one day told Miss Abby that she wanted to go to high school. As a result of Abby's tutoring and her own determination, Suzy was able to enter as a second year pupil and to maintain grades adequate for her to graduate. During that period she continued to live with Miss Abby and to assist her in various household tasks.

Miss Abby, proving herself to be more than an employer, took pleasure in directing a program of reading for her, making available many of the books from her own library.

Abby herself recently told me that she was convinced that reading for Suzy had become an avenue of escape from her painful past.

One day, Abby added, Suzy had asked her if she could visit the hospital where her baby had died. It was the first time she had referred to that time of her life. While at the hospital, she spoke with the Director of Nurses, recalling the night of her baby's death. It was as a result of her conversation with Miss MacD., emphasizing her interest in the care of babies and young children, that Suzy later was admitted as a member of the new class of nurses who would be living in a dormitory connected with the Good Shepherd Hospital.

Abby assured me that she intended to keep in close touch with Suzy. She further assured me that the hard work so far seemed to agree with the girl and that from reports she had received from Miss MacD., Suzy as a young student nurse was regarded by the staff as being energetic, trustworthy and capable.

Sept. 15, 1887

I was somewhat appalled to discover what Ted's idea of a bedroom-study is. He has succumbed to the latest fad among Uni-versity males to create a "Turkish Corner." He had a carpenter fashion a three-cornered couch-bed and covered it with a Turkish carpet and an array of bright colored pillows. There is a chair redone with some metallic woven stuff and an authentic Turkish prayer rug on the floor.

Set off on shelves and tables is a collection of brass decorations —tall pitchers, an authentic hookah, a curved dagger with carved handle, a fierce looking sword, a small opium pipe and an incense burner. Hanging on the wall is an ornately framed picture of a Turkish lady, a seductive look in her dark eyes, above the veiling that covers the rest of her face and torso. The table by his bed consists of a carved wooden tri-legged frame supporting a large hammered brass tray strewn with books, notebooks and a collection of pens and pencils. Situated under one uncurtained window is the only familiar piece of furniture—his old desk, littered with papers as always. And his second-hand typewriter.

He is writing for the *Onondagan* yearbook of the University and has joined the ranks of a fraternity—Delta Kappa Epsilon.

January 10, 1888

Tonight by moonlight I watched Teddy skate on the Canal from a spot where I was standing on the Clinton Street bridge by the Soldiers' and Sailors' Monument. If my words could flow as

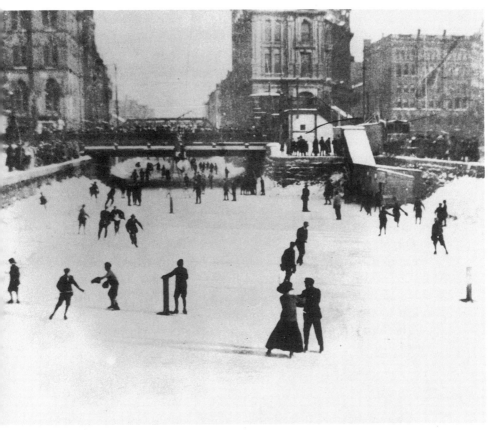

Skaters on the Erie Canal in the winter of 1888.
(Courtesy of The Erie Canal Museum)

easily as the coordinated muscles of his entire body responding to the rhythm of the music, I would give up doctoring and write poetry. Ted was actually dancing on the ice with young Molly O'Hearn as they practiced their figure eights together—their bright colored scarves whirling in cadence. With gloved fingers intertwined—Ted's left arm encircling her waist—they seemed to be flying together with the other laughing skaters as they disappeared down the dark frozen corridor of the Erie Canal.

March 16, 1888

By midnight Sunday, March 10, 1888, snow had fallen to such an extent that drifts had piled to the depth of ten feet and more in some sections of the city. On Monday morning all places of business and schools were closed. Trains, their engines buffeted by the blizzard, were stalled in the station yards. It was reported that 400 east-bound passengers were stranded here providing a bustling business for all the hotels. Hundreds of cattle were packed into freight cars along with twenty tons of mail. Over 200 horses were boarded temporarily in hotel stables. A patient of mine from Cazenovia who had been scheduled for admission to the hospital, was waylaid in Manlius. The stagecoach could not continue.

On March 14, 150 railroad laborers were transported from areas to the west to help shovel snow from the tracks and streets. In downtown Syracuse a horse-drawn snowplow careened to its side as it hit a drift on Genesee Street. The driver, badly hurt, was taken by ambulance to the hospital.

The blizzard was the worst one in the recorded history of the city.

April 30, 1888

A young matron, wife of an architect, recently came to me concerned about her menstrual problems and apparent inability to have a child. During the course of our conversation, she mentioned the time-consuming work of her husband who has come here as an assistant to Archimedes Russell, the much acclaimed Syracuse architect responsible for the planning and construction of many churches, fine homes and public buildings in Central New York. She spoke about her husband's interest in developing an artistic and achievable plan for this growing city by helping to choose architecture suitable for the needs of its people.

When I mentioned my own appreciation for the city's planting of shade trees along our own and other residential streets, she added that it is one of her husband's hopes to make this a beautiful city with planned areas for parks and play spaces for children. She explained that she and her husband had spent their honeymoon in Italy, had returned to this city determined to incorporate public water fountains and flower gardens within the parks such as had inspired them in Rome—not so ornate.

June 8, 1889

At Mrs. Coddington's funeral a few weeks ago I served as one of eight honorary women bearers. This was the first time in the city's history that women have been designated in that capacity. The funeral wreath was in place at the right hand side of the front door—its laquered black magnolia leaves intertwined with ivy announcing a death.

My friendship with Professor Coddington's wife has been one of long standing. Through her I have met many faculty members and their wives. And as her associate, being an active member of the Women's Alumnae Association, my acquaintance with other city women has greatly widened. My medical practice too has reflected my deeper involvement in the affairs of the community.

August 5, 1889

Mrs. Beatrice K. was in the office last week complaining of headache and severe back pain. She seemed inordinately worried. I asked her about how things were at home. She hesitated and then launched into a detailed description of a worsening problem between her husband and their thirteen-year-old son, John. "He beat the poor lad until his rump was black and blue. Yes, with his big hand—and then continued to slap him on the side of his head until the boy screamed." Mrs. K. caught my eye directly, her voice petulant, "What can I do? If I interfere he'll beat me." I asked what the son had done to cause such an outburst from his father. Apparently he had rebelled at being told to dispose of the garbage, a daily chore to which he had been assigned. The father complained that their kitchen smelled.

This mother is not the only one who has come to see me ostensibly to seek relief for a "headache." I have determined to use the subject of "Parents and Children" in a series of talks as part of this season's classes at the Y.W.C.A. The problems which surface over and over again is how to make the "punishment fit the crime" as we all deal with inevitable rebellious behavior of our emerging adolescent offspring. I have had ongoing experiences with my own son, Teddy.

October 16, 1890

The low-lying night-time clouds reflecting colors of brilliant red and yellow gave proof of the devasting fire that had enveloped the downtown area of the city including a leading hotel, the Leland House. Sounds of panic—fire-bells, the pounding of horses' hoofs, their frightened snorts, the intermittent screams of women, a perpetual siren blast, male voices shouting orders through bull horns.

Ted who had come to the house to have supper with us, quickly disappeared to join the growing crowd of spectators in order to be an on-site newspaper reporter.

Victims were being carried out on stretchers. Horse-drawn ambulances were there from both the hospitals with doctors on hand to give first aid. Police were doing their best to hold back the crowds and to cordon off affected areas so that firefighters could get their equipment as close as possible to the flames.

A couple horses became unmanageable—adding to the panic. Ted later reported that there was a shortage of water. Blankets and pillows were being thrown from the windows. There was terror on all sides. Besides the screaming women and frustrated men, the stench of smoke and fire spread over the city.

One woman jumped from the third floor of the hotel. A child

was being carried down a ladder. Walls crumbled. Tongues of fire shot upward. Crashing, crunching sounds. The acrid smell of smoke and burning human flesh. An actress, Cora Tanner, escaped from her room by sliding down a rope, finally being rescued by a life net spread out below.

I spent the entire night at the Good Shepherd Hospital doing whatever I could to help care for the more severely burned unfortunate victims. Six deaths resulted and there will be many victims suffering results of that fire for months afterward.*

January 30, 1891

Margaret Stanton,** a Syracuse College of Medicine graduate, class of '76, my friend and physician in town, had supper with me last evening. She told me about her year spent working and studying in England, France, Germany and Austria. How I envy her the experience! There have been many advances in scientific knowledge during the past few decades. Life expectancy both in Europe and here in the United States has been upgraded since the discovery that disease is spread by the presence of "germs." Especially important is the need for absolute cleanliness for obstetrical and surgical procedures. The names of Semmelweis in connection with childbed fever, of Pasteur's discovery of bacteria being the cause of infection, of Morton as the martyred discoverer of aenesthesia, of Lister as proponent of antisepsis in the operating room, of Koch's experiments with bacilli — Margaret spoke of these men as if they were old friends. In addition we now have

* Four years later, the nineteen mile pipeline bringing adequate water from Skaneateles Lake was finally completed, so that the city people had a safe drinking supply as well as a dependable fire-fighting source of water.

** Margaret Stanton, M.D., a member since 1878, served as treasurer of the Onondaga County Medical Society from 1888 until 1897. In 1898 she was elected vice-president and the following year became the first woman president of the Society. She was born in Syracuse December 20, 1844 and died in the same city January 22, 1903 great respect for Johns Hopkins Medical School in Baltimore, Md. and for its contribution to our profession of such fine physicians as William Welch, William Halsted, William Osler and Howard Kelly.

When Margaret was in London working at the Lying-in Hospital she mentioned that she often remembered the words of Dr. Oliver Wendell Holmes when he referred to the use of aenesthesia, "Now the fierce extremity of suffering has been steeped in the waters of forgetfulness." Margaret's experience took her beyond the walls of the hospital into the slums of London where she cared for many pregnant women whom she delivered in their proverty-stricken homes.

We talked until it was very late. We heard the old clock strike twelve.

May 17, 1892

Last evening an unusual event drew Margaret Stanton and me to the new Crouse College Auditorium at the University. A Bach organ recital. Unforgettable. The recently installed organ seemed to form an altar with the shining graduated pipes extending upward like huge candles to the carved wooden arch above the platform.

The entire Romanesque Revival structure of red sandstone standing atop University hill, is a tribute to its architect, Archimedes Russell, the Fine Arts Dean George Comfort and to the professors, the laborers and craftsmen, the University and the city of Syracuse itself.

Installed within the tower high above the four storied structure are the chimes, played each day at noon. The music of those chimes—inspiring to me—pervades the campus and surrounding vicinity at that hour.

March 18, 1893*
(two weeks after Inauguration of President Cleveland)

A recent letter from Ted in New York City tells of separate contact with three of his former Syracuse companions. Bill Stewart, his oldest friend, is studying at Medical School, now attached to Cornell University. Is getting instruction in the wards of New York Hospital and Bellevue. And last summer he had the opportunity of riding the ambulance. A far cry from picking wild strawberries in the field behind our house and selling newspapers on the corner of Salina Street.

One evening he went to visit his friend, Stephen Crane, who played baseball on the team at Syracuse University with Ted. Reportedly he is spending much of his time writing, observing the sordid life in the area around the Bowery, living in a boarding house with medical students, talking with old sailors and is befriending some of the prostitutes who hawk their wares along the Hudson River where freighters and old ships are at anchor. Ted says that this is the region of the city where he has gathered inspiration for his story, "Maggie, A Girl of the Streets"—just published and, unfortunately, not being very well received by the public.

One day during the spring he found another old friend, Elmer Sperry, in his New York office. After completing his engineering studies at Cornell he had spent some time in Chicago experimenting with electric arc lights and later actually invented a form of electric transmission device for street cars.

* The Financial Panic of 1893 swept the entire nation as a result of reckless railroad financing, unsound banking practices, unregulated interstate commerce and generalized labor strikes with widespread riots and bloodshed. On March 4, 1893 Grover Cleveland was inaugurated as President of the United States for his second term of office, previously having served as President from 1885 to 1889 when he won the election against Republican James G. Blaine. As a Democrat, his leadership was strong—supported by a similar majority in the Senate.

Grover Cleveland, son of Presbyterian minister Rev. Richard Cleveland, grew up in Fayetteville, N.Y. and was well-known in neighboring Manlius.

Lately he had been doing research on a method of sustaining stabilzation of moving objects based on an instrument called a "gyroscope." Ted was mightily impressed.

Ted apparently has been keeping himself busy working on newspaper assignments, ushering at night at various Broadway theaters and taking unimportant bit-parts on stage. It is an exciting life he would not have found in his hometown. Occasionally he sends us newspaper clippings as examples of his writing. Is keeping his sense of humor and seems to be constantly challenged and immersed in his new life.

In one way or another he consistently demonstrates his loyalty and affection to both Andrew and me.

January 16, 1894

Andrew and I sat quietly at home last evening enjoying the last warming embers of the hearth fire when there came a knock at the front door. I had been immersed in reading Oliver Wendell Holmes' "Autocrat of the Breakfast-Table." I brought myself back to reality, shook the wrinkles out of my dress and took off my new reading glasses before opening the front door. There stood my old friend and colleague, Doctor J. R. with his hat in his hand. "May I come in? In spite of the lateness of the hour?" He joined Andrew and me at the fireside.

He looked sharply at me, cleared his throat as he explained that he had just come from a long meeting of the Syracuse (City) Medical Society.* After having been in existence since 1847, finally tonight, January 16, 1894, the group voted to disband. Wide philosophical disunity within the ranks. There had been some harsh words. There was one faction which did not believe that women should be allowed within the society. Some members argued that women doctors would inevitably prove to be unac-

---

* The Onondaga County Medical Society, to which Millie has applied for membership and been duly denied, had been in continuous existence since 1806.

ceptable in this community. "Physiologically they are incapable of standing the strain. Intellectually they are unequal to men." Some believed that allowing women to become physicians threatened "the home and hearth of America" by ultimately diminishing the birth rate.

Faculty members, including Dr. John VanDuyn, and a few others had remained at the meeting after the final vote. This nucleus of city physicians and medical school professors had that evening decided to reorganize and support one another in forming a new Syracuse Academy of Medicine. He suggested with a kindly nod good night, that I should lose no time in seeking membership within the newly formed society.

At the end of two weeks, my application for membership was accepted. Under the name of Amelia Dann DeMott I am now, at the age of forty-seven, an active member and "Resident Fellow" of the newly established Syracuse Academy of Medcine whose purpose of existence is three-fold:

1. To cultivate and advance the Art and Science of Medicine
2. To promote Public Health
3. To maintain the honor, character and interests of the Medical profession.

Was it a long sought-for aura of victory that lifted me during my walk to the hospital this morning? I barely felt the sidewalk beneath my feet!

Jan. 15, 1896

Last year in 1895, in time for receiving the fall class, a new Medical School building was erected adjacent to the original structures. The four story red brick and limestone edifice was constructed to house lecture halls with tiered seating, faculty offices and medical library, laboratories, separate study rooms and lockers for men and women.

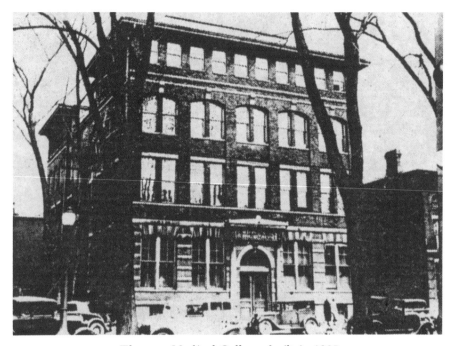

The new Medical College, built in 1895.

Specifications included 16-foot high ceilings, a ventilation stack extending from cellar to roof, large windows, steam radiators throughout the building, modern plumbing and an ice machine for cold storage. In addition to the laboratories, there were smaller lecture rooms and designated areas for storage. The anatomy room was outfitted with stone tables for cadaver dissection and overhung with electric lights. Anatomical charts and skeletal models lined the room and a separate area was equipped with marble wash basins. To enhance daytime visibility, skylights had been installed.

According the architect, Albert Brockway, new and progressive ideas had been incorporated into the plans after detailed study of similar medical buildings at Johns-Hopkins University, Columbia and Harvard.

The new students are lucky!

August 1, 1900

Andrew and I had been invited for tea at the Chancellor's home on Sunday. In my casual way of speaking I happened to mention that Andrew was looking forward to retirement from his business and that we were contemplating a move away from our College Place home near the campus so that Andrew could return to the life of a farmer. Chancellor Day looked a bit surprised and asked me what I was planning to do. I replied that at present I would continue practicing medicine, but that ultimately I would happily retire to being a farmer's wife.

The Chancellor then spoke about the growth of the University, how students from all walks of life are now studying here, how the Trustees have only recently proposed a plan to incorporate new blood into the Board membership. He added that in his opinion the board of Trustees should philosophically and actually reflect present day administrative and educational goals. Recently there has been talk of expanding courses of study at Syracuse University. The Board of Trustees should, he thought, represent the broadening interests of our student body. The information that Andrew, being a successful business man of the city about to retire to another way of life — agriculture — seemed to strike a responsive chord with the Chancellor.

September 15, 1900

Today Andrew received an invitation to become a member of the Syracuse University Board of Trustees. He has finally agreed to accept. I feel like shouting a silent hallelujah. Andrew, in his quiet reserved manner, will be an outspoken proponent of honesty, truth and fairness in all manner of University plans for

expansion. There has been discussion recently about a proposal
to establish a College of Agriculture here.

April 9, 1901

I shall feel few qualms or regrets as I finally plan to retire from
the practice of medicine. I look forward to spending many hours
with Andrew as we make mutual decisions concerning the new
house. During the process there is much for us to discover about
each other.

Ted decided several years ago to seek his fortune playing the
newspaper game in New York City: he writes that he is presently
busily established as a reporter for *The New York Sun*. I feel both
relieved and concerned. I realize it is high time for him to be on
his way. I wonder what is in store for him as he pursues his well-
developed propensity for seeking adventure. He seems to be in
love with his life of searching out newsworthy stories and discovering the allure of the theater both as a spectator and as an occasional stand-by actor.

I find myself daydreaming about the wife he will someday
marry and about finally seeing my unborn grandchildren. I avoid
the thought that Ted might establish a family far away from
Andrew and me. I have made up my mind that we shall probably
see him rarely during the next few yaers.

April 29, 1901

Ted recently enclosed the following account of a confrontation
that resulted from one of his first assignments.

> There has been one outstanding incident that made me
> realize I had no nose for news or else *The Sun* was not the great
> newspaper it was reputed to be. Daniel Kellogg, the city editor,
> the other day handed me a 'dead dog' assignment, information
> having come through customary sources for the gathering of

news—'dead dog with pups in a vacant lot away uptown.'

It seemed to me like one of those 'kidding' assignments the older staff men like to put up for the cubs. From my viewpoint there was no possible news in it. My opinion was confirmed when I assured myself that none of the other papers were paying any attention to the report of a dead dog with pups. However I did discover that there were six motherless puppies in the process of being adopted by a nervous goose. The sob story had first-page distinction and was printed word for word as I had written it.

Julian Ralph, the preeminent star of the staff, stopped at my desk to reassure me that the dead dog and goose yarn was a typical *Sun* story. I contended there was no news in the item and that in my estimation the *Sun* was a NEWSPAPER. Anything unusual, Ralph assured me, was news.

The thought came to me that a dead dog in the environs of Solvay would not be regarded as first-page news by the newspaper editors of Syracuse. The story excited comment inside the office and out. It must have been news after all. Then and there I concluded that I had no news sense. Later I learned about the *Sun's* fondness for unusual animal stories.

September 14, 1901

President William McKinley died today after being shot on September 6 while he was in Buffalo. Vice-president Theodore Roosevelt, another Republican, becomes our twenty-sixth President having been sworn in today.

What with the Cuban situation, upheaval in Europe and strikes in this country, conversation at our house is never dull.

February 11, 1902

Recently I had an urgent call to visit a former patient of mine, Mrs. McC., who now lives on East Jefferson Street. She lay in bed shaking with chills and fever. Her sister, Evelyn, a nurse, who was caring for her for five days reported that she had been having diarrhea and coughing with spasms of pain in her chest. Refused all food. Following examination of her lungs I diagnosed her illness as pneumonia. Advised continued bed-rest, cool alcohol rubs alternated with hot compresses to her chest, soft foods as she was able to tolerate them and as much water as she could drink. I encouraged her sister to continue with the good nursing care and to keep the children away from the sick-room. I expect her to pass the crisis within a day or two.

As I was packing up my bag to leave I became conscious of a child's muffled cry. Nurse Evelyn pointedly avoided answering my question when I inquired about the cry which seemed to come from a closed door off the patient's bedroom. When the cry became a scream Miss Evelyn opened the door of a dark closet where a three-year-old girl with tousled brown hair was standing in her crib yelling at the top of her voice. Miss E. lifted her from her feces-stained mattress, wrapped her snugly in a blanket and mumbled baby-talk words until the child stopped sobbing. I followed them down the stairs to the parlor, but before I left the house at the front door I felt the child's forehead.

Instinctively I folded back the blanket, could see that the child was undernourished, pale, eyes blinking from exposure to the sunny room. As I proceeded to remove the soiled sweater I noticed the stumped malformation of her left arm and dangling hand. The little hand had webbed fingers with a sixth finger imperfectly developed.

Miss E. was quick now to speak up. "It's all right, Doctor. She was born that way and she can't talk either. Her Mother keeps her in the closet so that people won't see her. I know she feels terrible about it because it's her fault. You see she sinned while she was carrying the baby. She knows she's to blame. Even the Priest can't seem to help her."

Yesterday I spoke to Dr. M about the case. He had heard of such occurrences and wants to examine the baby. He is sure he can correct the webbed finger condition and remove the supernumerary digit, but physical and emotional restitution of the child herself is another matter. Whatever happens I want to follow through on the care of this unfortunate baby girl and her Mother.

Mrs. McC's pneumonia is only minor to her own total recovery.

April 10, 1903

It has come to my attention that there are a growing number of foreign students on our campus chiefly from Asian countries. I would like to encourage certain of these students to be invited to speak at the University Alumnae gatherings and especially at Syracuse Women's Congress* whose purpose is to keep its fifty members abreast of worldwide events especially affecting women. I should like to promote communication with certain of these students after they have returned to their various home countries. I will.

August 10, 1903

Andrew has been looking for some time for appropriate land to buy in the area of Syracuse. When the time comes for his retirement, he would like nothing better than to have a farm. Since he grew up on his own father's farm in the north country, he has dreamed of returning to the "land." Last Sunday we drove four miles out on Genesee Street on the road to Fayetteville. There Andrew pointed out a place he is genuinely interested in. Apparently the present owner is old and too feeble to continue the work. His sons have moved away and are far from interested in pursuing the work a farm demands. So he and his wife have determined to sell out. There is a ramshackle old farmhouse, a barn needing a great deal of repair as well as various other out-buildings. At the present time if we do buy it we would do nothing except to raze

* At that time Millie was as office-holding member of both organizations.

the existing house.

There are several neglected fruit orchards — apple, pear and plum. Land which has obivously been ploughed and planted for years seems to Andrew to be spent. Much work will be required to re-establish fertility and productivity to the acreage. The challenge lights up Andrew's whole being. I surmise he will ultimately make the investment, especially if he can persuade Ted to go into his downtown Empire Metal Company business with him. We shall certainly continue to live on College Place across from the University until the time comes for us to move finally to the farm wherever it ultimately may be located. And there is no doubt in my mind that I shall continue to practice medicine. My patients are my friends — most of them. I cannot relinquish my obligation to them until we both decide to retire.

November 1, 1903

I have noticed a paucity of entries in my Journal lately. Understandable — even to a stranger who might someday peruse these jottings of incidents and reports. I may one of these days after my retirement have time to read over some of the events I wrote down those many years ago. I might glean some perspective on my life.

Of course both my time and energy have been spent this year in seeing old patients and admitting new ones, helping them when I could to deal with an increasing variety of problems.

I have spent a number of evening hours as well with the young women on campus who have been eager to establish their new Greek sorority — being cautious not to make initial decisions they may later regret, to help them write their purpose clearly and understandably and to plan for their future growth. Together we have had meetings with Bishop Huntington and the acting Dean of Women. I have offered our present home on College Place for informal discussions. I like the young ladies. They are, as a group, serious, above-average students, unsophisticated but not naive, appreciative of humor and eager to present themselves well on campus. During the process of organization we have come to know and understand one another surprisingly well.

November 15, 1903

Edith Hodgeson who has come to work for us, continues her faithful services, so that I need not be concerned with keeping the pantry cupboards stocked.

There are days when I cannot find time to read the newspaper, although through Andrew I am kept abreast of politics. And, to boot, I know more about the stock market and the fluctuating cost of metals than I ever knew or cared to know before.

Ted stops in now and then when he comes to town to see his special friend, Miss Helen B. Of course we do catch occasional short glimpses of him when he manages a fleeting hello and good bye.

Andrew and I have decided to purchase the farm!

December 14, 1903

Andrew will soon be involved in preparation of the ground for situating the new house and for planting a garden. He has already spoken to Albert Brockway, the architect whose work we both admire. It was he who drew up plans for the new medical school —a fine example of his ability to combine fitness of function with the art of architectural design.

I like to picture in my mind a red brick colonial house where we will welcome family and friends—a home with aspects of a farm-house where food from the garden and orchard can be stored, prepared and shared.

I can already see a den with a fireplace—wood crackling—a room where we shall spend much time together, where I can read in my old comfortable chair by the window with orientation to the west, where my desk and a bookcase can be at hand because I plan to do considerable catching up on long overdue reading and writing. And there will be a leather covered couch where Andrew can rest after long hours of work in his garden. And of course his card table and his old Windsor chair will be there too.

I want a house large enough for hospitable entertainment of neighbors and friends with at least two comfortable guest rooms and a room and bath for Edith. I want safe play space for grandchildren and an accessible toy cupboard. I hope there will be many children. And in the dining room I want a swinging door to the kitchen, wood wall paneling and a plate rail! And a niche for the grandfather's clock.

"Such stuff as dreams are made of!"

March 5, 1904

Last week I met with Bishop H. at the Rectory. Because of his interest in the establishment and ongoing direction of affairs at the Good Shepherd Hospital, I have on many previous occasions talked with him. This time he wanted to discuss another concern. Although there are already seven sororities established on the University Campus he has concluded that there is still too much loneliness and lack of direction among many young women on the campus. He sees a need for more women to live together in a real house—not a dormitory—where close friendships can readily flourish, where mutual support on all levels can be sponsored, where a mother figure could direct the maintenance of the living quarters. The Bishop has already been involved in helping several groups of young women to inaugurate possible "sororities" with chapters on this campus. He asked for my help in meeting with one group of fifteen enthusiastic undergraduates as they formulate their plans to establish the Alpha chapter of Alpha Gamma Delta as the eighth sorority to be established on the Syracuse Campus. One of their aims will be to promote top scholarship. I shall be glad to spend time with this particular group of students.

April 15, 1904

I have become lately aware of a disturbing situation affecting certain members within our own medical community. One well-known and respected Syracuse physician has died of self-induced morphine poisoning. It has been generally accepted as fact that he was often in severe pain from rheumatism and since his wife died last year he had tended to remain aloof from even his best friends. In spite of his infirmity he has been faithful in caring for his many patients and generally appeared in good spirits, gradually seeming to recover from the loss of his Mary. It was with shock that his son discovered the slumped body in his office with clear evidence that he had purposefully overdosed himself with an injection of morphine.

We now have been alerted to the practice of drug addiction not only on the part of physicians themselves, but among our patients —many of whom have depended on acquiring narcotics through mail-order. Proprietary medicines (sold by the owner of the patent, formula or brand name) can be purchased at almost any store. Frequently these so-called cures contain morphine, cocaine or heroine. Even the soothing syrup sold for babies may contain opium.

Spring Tonics said to alleviate "indigestion, headache, fever, back pain, weariness and catarrh" often contain as high as 44% alcohol. Lydia Pinkham's famous Vegetable Compound, advertised widely in newspapers contains not only esoteric herbs but 21% alcohol.

Through articles appearing in magazines, lectures given before women's clubs and educational efforts of the American Medical Society, there has developed a public demand for curtailment of the patent medicine trade. Proposal has been made in Congress for future enactment of a fedral act to insure the sale of Pure Food and Drugs. It is high time. "Bottled Quackery" has already caused unnecessary deaths in this country from cancer, kidney disease and tuberculosis.

September 10, 1904

At the end of a long afternoon of seeing patients, Barbara came quietly into my office announcing that there were still two young women waiting to see me — without appointment. She proceeded to usher into my consultation office two nuns dressed in full starched white headdress and flowing black habit. They sat prim and silent, bowing slightly toward me as I entered the room. The younger of the two rose, held out her hand to me, introduced her friend, Sister Jenny. It was only then with a flash of recognition that I realized I was addressing Suzy who smiled rather shyly at me.

"Doctor DeMott," she said, "I know you are surprised to see me after so many years, but I shall not take much of your time. I have written a letter for you. I have it here. I have much to tell you. I have written the letter so that you will, I hope, understand my long silence. I have always been grateful to you for what you have done for me." She spoke as if the lines were from a play — pale words.

I noted a darting, seeking expression in Suzy's eyes that belied her nun-calm demeanor. Her eyes seemed almost electrified as she handed me the letter. The nun's habit had not only concealed the envelope, but had physically hindered me from coming close to the human being wearing it. I felt unable to say anything appropriate to the moment as I took Suzy's hand-written offering without touching her.

I simply spoke in my usual professional tone of voice thanking her and her friend for their visit as I accompanied them to the front door.

Somehow is a strange way, I sensed that Suzy's visit to my office was once again a call for help. This time she was coming not as a troubled child, not as a prostitute, not as a rebellious young mother, not as a poor sick cast-off from society but as a Nun — an experienced nurse of the Order of St. Francis — a dignified member of the staff of St. Joseph's Hospital. I was puzzled.

I read her long letter describing her life as a novitiate, her period of instruction—both religious and academic—the long arduous experience she had undergone, the mystical and spiritual happiness she had derived from the hard work, the discipline and finally the fear she expressed that in spite of her repeated confessions and appropriate penances performed, she felt that she was still not truly worthy of belonging to the Franciscan Order and her adopted hospital community. The guilt she still bore from her pre-baptismal transgressions had surfaced with vengeance—now weighed heavily.

The old Suzy, with remarkable determination, has become a woman. I am in awe of her accomplishments. Yet, here she is again appealing to me for help. What untapped means of healing could I release? How can I possibly give hope to this Franciscan nun whose need, I know, is to rid herself of the guilt brought on by prostitution and her long-denied responsibility for the death of her unwanted child?

———————————————

To retire from the active practice of medicine next year is becoming for me mandatory. Andrew too has been busier than ever at his factory this year. He has taken on a new man who will be spending most of his time on the road making necessary calls on customers.

With the new house already in the process of construction, Andrew spends hours supervising the supervisor. So all in all, for both of us, this has been a demanding year—demanding of our ability to adapt not only to each other but to the changing needs of each day as it dawns.

December 22, 1904

My entries during this entire year have been fewer than almost any year since I began to write in this journal. Not surprising.

I have been overwhelmed with the details of my new domestic

role. Never in my life before have I been imposed on as I have been this year! I have had to choose wall paper, decide the color of paint to be used, designate this or that material to be used for reupholstering the old furniture. Andrew leaves the department of interior management entirely up to me. I close my eyes at night with colors and designs flashing in my brain.

This year I have also been called upon to invest my energy into University affairs by getting myself enmeshed in Women Alumnae Association, becoming president of a Current Events Discussion group, backing the Red Cross Chapter in the city and lending my support to Women's Rights locally. Internationally, the papers are full of Japan's recent attack on Russia and what it may portend in Europe.

Suzy's letter when I finally found uninterrupted time to read it, explained in decorous detail the course of the five years she had spent in preparation for being fully accepted as a Franciscan nun within the Roman Catholic Church. During those five years she was not allowed to serve in the hospital as a nurse. After the first nine months of devotion, study and religious training she promised before the altar to become a faithful Bride of Christ and the church. She, with Jenny and the other young women who made the promise together, wore traditional white wedding apparel.

Becoming a Postulant during the second year, Suzy gave herself unstintedly to the Church and its Community, devoting her time and energy to more study and to the obedient performance of menial domestic tasks.

As a Novice she then began a third year, one designed for periods of absolute silence. Being forbidden to speak during long hours of meditation, she learned the meaning of prayer and total devotion to the spiritual life.

During the fourth year, wearing the traditional black nun's robe and white headdress, she was once again allowed to speak to co-workers as she performed the many arduous tasks assigned to her. This portion of her preparation, Suzy admitted, was a year of struggle as she dealt with doubts, questions relating to morality and her own rebellious instincts.

Finally she earned the right to wear the authentic Franciscan nun's habit. Hung about her neck was a heavy metal cross and encircling her waist was a twisted black cord tied with three knots —symbols of her vow to live a life of poverty, chastity and obedience.

Once more after five years of preparation, testing and idealistic anticipation, Suzy returned for service to the sick and dying as a nurse at the hospital. Jenny remained her close friend and confidant throughout the years of study and training as the two young women together earned the Franciscan right to return to their profession.

To the best of my ability I shall respond to her letter. I must also let her know of my imminent plans to retire.

September 19, 1904

As I was about to close the office late yesterday afternoon Andrew stopped in asking me to drive with him to take a look at the farm. He has had a crew of men tearing down the old house and barn—wanted to see what progress they had made. Old gray Rex seemed hell-bent to get us there and back. Got his blood circulating—and ours too.

The walls of the farmhouse are all down. A tremendous clean-up job ahead. Only the old brick chimney still stands—dangerously askew. The men have cleaned out the barn, piled up old hay and debris. A massive bonfire is scheduled for tomorrow if the wind calms down.

December 26, 1904

This morning I had a telephone call from Sister Superior at the hospital. With saddened voice she notified me that Sister Susan Mary was extremely ill—that she had asked to see me.

Briefly she explained that Sister has been in charge of the sick

baby nursery on night duty. About two o'clock this morning Sister
Susan Mary had called her, seemed distraught because of the sudden and unexpected death of one of the tiny babies under her
care. She had called the Night Supervisor as well as the Chaplain
whom she had roused from sleep. They had both come to her
assistance. By seven-thirty a.m. she had retired to her own room,
as was her custom.

Some time during the afternoon Sister Jenny had gone to her
friend's room. As there came no response to her knock she quietly
opened the unlocked door. Sister Superior's voice broke with a
sob. "Doctor, Sister Susan has attempted suicide. Using small
sharp-pointed scissors from her sewing basket Sister Susan Mary
was successful in severing the jugular vein at the left side of the
neck! First aid on the part of her friend has saved our Sister's life."

With no delay I headed for St. Joseph's Hospital. A nurse
escorted me to her room where Suzy was recovering from shock
and loss of blood—pale, eyes closed, exhausted. The Chaplain
had just finished administering the Last Rites of the Church and
now there was absolute quiet in the room. I held Suzy's hand,
squeezed it as I spoke a few gentle words to her. The Chaplain
and the nurse left Suzy and me alone in the room. As she slept I
continued to sit silently by her bedside still holding her hand.
Some time later when she waked, she turned her head toward me,
smiled a tremulous smile and with an expression of love I have
never seen before, Suzy spoke with faltering words. "Doctor — I
know — that — you know — what I know. — Only you. — Help
me. Please help me."

I comforted her as best I could, saying that as soon as she felt
able I would see her in my office, that we would then talk about
many things. After half a life-time of searching for absolution
Suzy has suffered a final attempt to deliver herself as a fitting
sacrifice. Shall I ever be able help her explain that "black hole" in
her mind so that she will be freed to go on with the good life she
has found? How can I help her to forgive herself?

Suzy will, I am sure, ultimately deal with the guilt that has almost killed her. She will discover strength acquired through her latest suffering. The fact of her survival has been a revelation to her. She can live to overcome future adversities.

Soon, I am confident, that by remaining within the protective shelter of the Church, her ability to cope with inevitable joys and sorrows at the hospital will broaden. She must recognize that she is no longer "a sinner." The time has come for Suzy to forgive herself. By so doing she will free herself to live the useful life she has chosen with deep faith in her religion and growing confidence in herself.

I shall never forget Suzy.

January 1, 1905

I have witnessed many changes in this city since my teaching days of the 1870's. There is one item of special interest to me — the population of this city has tripled. Many babies have been born. More children are now surviving illnesses that caused their deaths a few decades ago.

Instead of the salt industry being foremost among our industries, today the city is noted for its manufacture of bicycles, typewriters, automobiles, steel and chemicals. It has become a center for distribution of agricultural products, manufactured goods and machinery, as well as being a crossroad for human transportation — east, west, north and south. The New York Central Railroad tracks run directly through our downtown district! We are noted for that phenomenon along with the adjacent line-up of saloons, dance halls and flop houses.

The business areas have grown with the building of the County Court House, the new City Hall, the Andrew Carnegie Public Library, our Syracuse University College of Physicians and Surgeons as well as the newly constructed hotels, churches, banks, department stores and schools.

From the hills overlooking the city stand the numerous buildings of the University, the hospitals and stately homes. I find myself being amazed at the changes in the skyline of the city as I look toward Onondaga Lake from East Genesee Street hill.

Architectural design reflects the countries of origin of the people who have come here to make their homes. There are scattered examples of building, details of which may have originated in England, France, Holland, Italy, Germany or Spain — not to mention the Greek Revival style homes, Gothic cottages and cobblestone houses to be seen in outlying towns or along the country roads of the County. The plan of our streets, the park areas, the fountains, our gardens often remind visitors of our European origins. Even the name of our city of Syracuse commemorates a city built before the time of Christ by the Corinthians on the island of Sicily — Siracusa.

Over the years, city government has developed in response to the need of serving our fast growing population. The importance of the Mayor and the elected City Council has increased as has the influence of various Commissions — Education, Public Health, Fire Prevention, Sanitation, Water, Parks and Recreation. All have taken on new significance since my medical practice began in 1878.

And now this city, because of its geographic location forming a hub on an axis plumb in the center of New York State, attracts conventions, conferences, political rallies, religious revivals, itinerant entertainment — even the coming to town of the circus, sports competitions as well as the annual State Fair. And of course, traveling salesmen.

Crime has increased. Robberies, "body-snatching" by grave-diggers, pick-pocketing, prostitution, shop-lifting, and occassional murder, drunkeness. Our jails are often full to capacity. The courts on all levels have been kept busy.

Automobiles are being seen more and more on our streets. Franklin cars are now manufactured here. Streetcar tracks have been laid, some now being run by power derived from overhead electric cables. I am especially gratified to see the streets well lit at night now that we are launched into the twentieth century.

Between the time of the Civil War, when as a young girl I lived
in Manlius to the present time as I prepare to retire from the
practice of medicine in Syracuse, woman-kind has been caught
up in periodical high winds of political, domestic, religious and
cultural turmoil. Although I have not been at the forefront of the
movement for women's rights I have felt the strong impact of
prejudice: as a female medical student, as a practicing physician
chiefly concerned with the diseases and plights of women, as a
Mother of a fatherless son, as one seeking admission to professional societies and as an avid reader of medical journals,
newspapers and popular literature as well.

Important changes began to appear in 1848 when a few serious-
minded women met together in the home of Elizabeth Cady Stanton in the small town of Seneca Falls in Upstate New York. Their
concerns were the rights of women, the condition of Negroes in
slavery and the involvement of women in the Temperance Movement. As a result, the first Women's Rights Convention met in
Syracuse in 1852.

Slowly women have been acquiring a voice in public affairs. By
1890 two separate women's rights associations active in different
portions of the country joined together to form a National American Suffrage Association with top leaders being Elizabeth Cady
Stanton, Susan B. Anthony, Lucy Stone, Matilda Joslyn Gage
and others from various locations within the United States. With
the additional help from prominient men—clergymen, politi-
cians, newspaper editorialists, playwrights and lecturers—I hope
that sufficient effort has finally been gathered to ensure passage
of an Amendment to the U.S. Constitution giving women the
right to vote.

I have attended many lectures myself by women—each promoting her own individual philosophy on women's rights. The
first was back at the time I lived in Kirkville in the 1870's when
Matilda Gage from nearby Fayetteville came to speak at our
Union Church. There were others over the years including Victoria Claffin Woodhull who had come from the mid-west as a

strong advocate of faith healing and free love. Most clearly I remember the words of Elizabeth Cady Stanton, her daughter Lucy Stone and Susan Anthony.

After my retirement I hope to have more time to spend on promoting the ongoing advancement of women's suffrage.

January 5, 1905

Native Indians lived here long before the White Man even dreamed of settling in our beautiful valley. I was reminded of this last week when a young Indian who has done some carpentry work for me asked if I would go to the nearby Onondaga Indian Reservation to visit his grandmother who was very ill. I questioned him about the "Medicine Man" who sometimes cares for the sick on the Reservation. He scowled, hinted that the "so-called doctor there" dealt in magic potions, mixed various herbs as medicine. He no longer trusts the "Medicine Man." Said his grandmother has grown much worse. If I would come, he would accompany me to show me where she lives. I finally agreed to go with him.

We hitched up old Rex and together drove along the dirt road south to the Reservation which I had never before visited.

We found "Nomah," young David's grandmother, huddled under a bright colored, hand woven blanket asleep on her bed in a little cabin near the Longhouse. Indeed she was very ill. When he woke her, David explained in words she understood that he had brought a lady doctor from the city to help her get rid of her pain. She looked at me with a sad, but patient expression, murmured a few words to David in her native tongue.

As I pulled back the covers I could see that she was emaciated, dehydrated and extremely weak. My hand on her forehead told me of her fever. Another Indian—David's father—appearing at the cabin door, bowed politely to me. He then explained to me that the following day they would, according to his mother's wish, carry her to the woods where they would lay her on a bed of pine needles at the foot of an old oak tree, carefully cover her with her blanket, speak an Indian prayer of farewell and leave her alone until the Great Spirit would come for her.

I left David quietly weeping at her side. With Rex trotting along at an easy pace my drive back to the city was strangely comforting — a time for reverie — to comtemplate the wisdom of our native Indians and to determine to learn more about their history and customs.

January 15, 1905

To comprehend the advances in medicine since my confinement in the Pest Hole when I was fighting the deadly forces of typhoid fever during the summer of 1875, I must stretch my mind over the years into the beginning of this new twentieth century. Long before the establishment of medical schools at Harvard, Chicago, Philadelphia, Johns Hopkins at Baltimore and our own at Syracuse University, the training of medical students in this country was attained through preceptorships. A *man* arranged with an older physician to become his Preceptor. The agreement might involve three years of study centered in the practitioner's office. Also in New York State the young man was expected to attend two full courses of bona fide medical lectures of 16 weeks each, study the doctor's textbooks, make himself useful in the office, learn to mix medicines and tinctures, greet patients in a professional manner, make certain housecalls with the older man, study diagnosis at the bedside under the guidance of his mentor, learn proper remedies and how to prescribe them, write a thesis on some medical subject, pass an oral examination before a Board of Censors, have attained at least the age of 21 years and be of good moral character. The State then might at that point award him a license to practice medicine.

Now women with proper accreditation are finally being accepted at a few of our university medical schools. Progress has been slow.

In the field of Public Health we have learned the reasons for providing pure water and milk for our people, how to promote educational means and adequate methods of preventing disease, to make wide use of our knowledge of immunization and antisepsis. Diphtheria, tetanus, hydrophobia and smallpox *can* now be prevented. Deaths and serious complications continue from measles, scarlet fever, meningitis. From the days of routine bloodletting to treat disease, attitudes and methods of treatment have radically improved.

Surgical techniques have advanced. Hospitals are no longer regarded as "death houses." Treatment of the insane now involves hope for improvement. Babies are surviving their first years of life. Mothers no longer fear puerperal fever. Ambulances can be depended upon when necessary to carry the critically ill or injured to hospitals for immediate care. A growing number of our promising young women are being trained to be nurses in those hospitals as well as to make visits to patients in their home under the aegis of the Visiting Nurses Association, established as a private agency in Syracuse in 1890.

I now have a telephone both at home and in my office. We have electric lights. Our garbage and trash is collected. We have central heating and inside plumbing in town. Our main laboratories are equipped with microscopes as well as with finely calibrated measuring devices and with diagnostic aids of all sorts. Electronic instruments of various sorts are beginning to appear in our hospitals—useful for both diagnosis and treatment. The practice of medicine has changed drastically. Let a skeptic read the minutes of the Medical Society and the Academy as well!

January 20, 1905

For many years I have performed a minor ritual of winding the old grandfather clock. Last Sunday evening that ritual became a time of contemplation for me. I was thinking in retrospect of the life I have been privileged to live during the past thirty years and now the new life I am about to enter at the age of sixty. As the clock marked off the minutes with its ticking beats I was pulled further into my reverie of time as I checked the old clock's historic view of human life: a small infinity within this family of mine. Birth, growth, adaptation, aging, death—hour to hour, day to day, month to month, year to year.

We shall take this family clock with us to the new red brick house. It will oversee our new life—Andrew's and mine. It will witness the coming and going of many people in and out of unlocked doors. Now I have decided exactly where we shall place it—the corner of the stair landing so that anyone can tell the time from upstairs or downstairs or as we pass it midway. Its chimes will alert us no matter where we are within the house.

Unconsciously both Andrew and I have been working year in and year out for this time of our lives to arrive. And it has.

January 23, 1905

Tonight I am focussing on this Journal of mine. This will be my last entry in it. The Journal reflects many changes in my life as a woman physician since I began it almost thirty years ago—it records not only the scheduled humdrum of daily happenings, but it has become a measure of my own personal fluctuating array of sensations—the eagerness of youth, motherhood, fervor, the loss of my parents, grief, readjustment, meeting the exigencies of the moment, vulnerability, doubt, wonderment, spiritual growth, ultimate recognition of my own strengths and frailties.

I am about to retire from the life of a nineteenth century woman who had the timerity to become a physician, now to take up with anticipation a brand new specialty—that of being my Andrew's full-time wife.

And so this long sporadic Journal comes to an inevitable end.

PART III

Millie's Second Marriage, Retirement,
Community Service, Travel and
Granddaughter's Memories

PART III

During the interim, between the time of Millie's retirement from the practice of medicine to the time when she became a grandmother, there were significant events taking place on East Genesee Street hill.

The red brick house became a reality. Furnishings retained from her parents' farmhouse—chairs, tables, beds, chests of drawers—were refinished. The old grandfather's clock found its new niche. Velvet hangings and new draperies were purchased. Oriental rugs covered the hardwood floors. An oak and brown leather divan with Mission rocking chair, a desk, Windsor chairs and small tables furnished the den, one wall of which was lined with books. In the corner fireplace, brass andirons supported a huge pile of firewood ready to warm the room.

A vegetable garden was planted behind the old apple orchard. A flower bed was planned. Shrubbery softened the lines of the pillared entrance-way. Sidewalks were installed. The old maple trees in the front yard were pruned, their wide branches already offering shade in front of the red brick house.

Ted decided against becoming a Paris foreign correspondent for the *New York Herald* and instead agreed to return to Syracuse to be assistant manager at Grandfather DeMott's factory. Ted married his old time love, Helen Bowers—my Mother—and began to oversee the construction of their new home, a gray stone house situated next to his parents with only a gravel driveway separating the two on the crest of East Genesee Street hill. More fruit trees were planted—pear, peach and plum. Under the

167

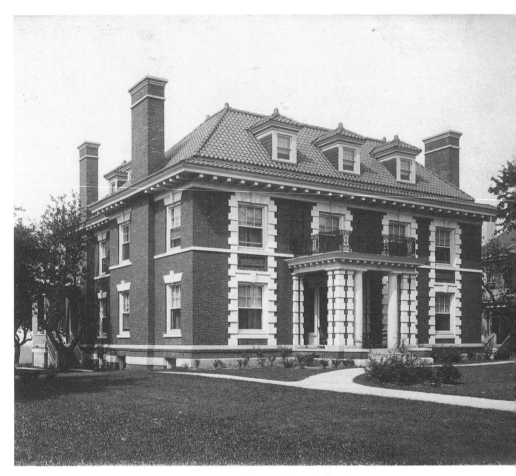

The Red Brick House.

talented direction of my Mother their new house was furnished —
a home readied for another generation of central New York children.

As far back as I can remember I felt as comfortable in my
Grandparents' home as I felt within my own parents' house. The
doors of the big red brick house were never locked, so that standing as it did across the driveway from our house, it became a safe
haven for me always. Every cranny was mine to explore from the
dark dankness of the cellar to the mysteries of the attic.

Early in childhood a close bond began to develop between my
Grandmother and me — a bond destined to become strong and
firm. Memories now seem kaleidoscopic — images, sounds, smells,
sensations provide minimal sequence in recall. A word, a tone, a
fragrance evokes another vignette. Present reality recedes. Colors
and images blur, then clarify into sharp outline and feature. One
after the other. Sensations too — love, hate, awe, ecstacy, quan-
dary, sudden revelation — play one upon the other.

Millie, M.D., as I write about her, releases herself from the
past and invites me to glimpse into her mind, her heart, to sense
her vital spark. As she does so, she provides me with unexpected
insight through which to view myself as I was growing up.

The great-great-great grandfather's clock standing in the corner of my own dining room has been ticking away generational
gaps. Hand-constructed from cherry wood by an unknown fore-
bear, the timepiece fits snugly from floor to ceiling into the corner. The often repaired mechanism, still empowered by a worn
brass key, synchronizes the rotation of hands with the rhythmic
swinging of the pendulum. A metal plaque clearly but crudely
etched is firmly fastened above the pendant disc, verifying the
date of completion — June 1817.

The clock's face is cracked and discolored but still preserved
above the Roman numeralled hour of twelve in its framed oval is
painted a seascape in miniature. A sailboat, its white canvas bal-

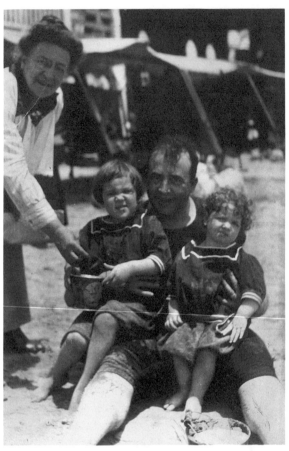

At Atlantic City beach.

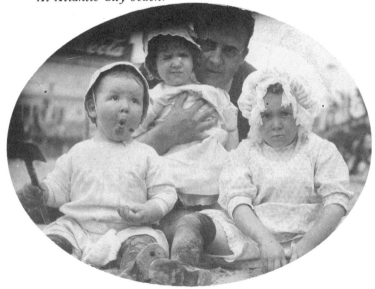

Playing with our Dad.

looning, seems to whip around a promontory where, as sentinel, a little church has stood these many years. When the long glass door of the casement is ajar, a message tacked to the rough wood inside comes to light. On brown crumbling paper a poem is barely legible:

> I am a clock as my face appears.
> I have walked on time for a hundred years.
> Many men have fallen since my life began;
> Many will fall ere my span is done.
> I have buried the world with its hopes and fears
> In my long, long walk of revolving years.

Time merges from dawn to noon to night, as spring follows winter and fall follows after summer year after year. Children's laughter and squabbles, the deeper tones of their elders — serious or flippant — repetitive birthday chanting and the babble of table talk has blended and blurred with the familiar ticking - ticking.

During the passage of almost twenty years, the period that over-lapped our lives — her last and my first — the clock kept time as a revered piece of furniture in my Grandmother's home. Although the chimes were silenced long ago, one vibrant tone continues to denote thirty minutes past each hour.

My Grandmother used to strum the guitar and sing in a sort of conversational tone the same songs she had sung as a third, fourth and fifth grade teacher many years before. She liked being a teacher. One time when I begged her to play we discovered a mouse and her brood of tiny bare wiggly babies in a nest beneath the strings of her guitar. I remember the high squeaking sound they made, the pinkness of them. A wonder it was that Dinah, her black cat, had not found this family of mice.

On other occasions my Grandmother sat patiently beside me at her desk as I learned to copy headlines from the morning newspaper. Soon I would be able to read simple words and sentences. She taught me to count and to recognize numbers. I learned colors reflected from a many-faceted crystal hung in a sunny window. I remember running about the room as I tried to catch the darting colors—much to my Grandmother's amusement and encouragement.

I remember one fall on a rainy day as the yellow leaves swirled in eddying circles on the front lawn. We were upstairs in her sewing room. She was darning a hole in my Grandfather's sock as I sat at her knee on the floor playing a favorite game with buttons. Dumping them all together from a brown leather pouch onto a tin tray, I liked to sort them, matching colors and sizes.

I liked to feel the texture of them—the hard ones, the carved ones, the sparkly ones, the soft velvety ones, the tiny ones that stuck to my finger. Some of them I strung onto a strong linen thread and wore as beads around my neck.

"Will you tell me a story?" I asked her as I looked up into her wrinkled face. She smiled and said she would tell me about a soldier who had fought in a war called the American Revolution. His name was Jonathan and he had been wounded in battle. He had been hit by a bullet and had been lying for more than an hour unconscious on the battlefield at Lexington, Massachusetts. Finally when he was able to open his eyes he could feel a fierce pain in his leg.

Blood had flowed, had oozed and clotted. Flies had laid their eggs in the wound. He knew there would be an infection if he did not act quickly. So, she went on, he raised himself on his elbow, found his sharp pocket knife and with clenched teeth, cut a deep furrow around the wound where flies had settled. Taking a deep breath he dug out the bullet and wiped away the dirt and blood. With another deep breath he stuffed his handkerchief into the hole, fell back onto the battlefield and fainted. I watched dumbfounded as my Grandmother acted out the part of the soldier who

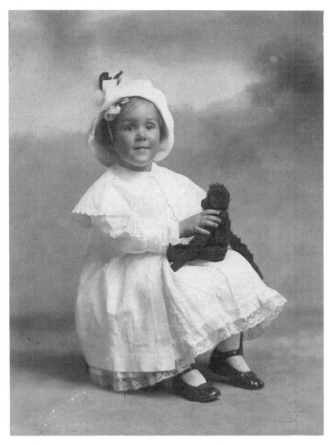

Honney with her monkey, Jocko, after packing Ophelia into a trunk for a round-the-world trip with Grandmother.

had saved his own life. He was, she explained, a "survivor."

That was a true story about one of my Grandmother's ancestors and, as she indicated "one of your ancestors too." Before that day I had not known about ancestors or survivors. "Tell-me-a-story" became like a chorus throughout our many, many conversations.

———————

Daily there were new experiences for me as the oldest child in a
growing family, no matter whether at school or at church or
dancing school. She encouraged me to be forthright in whatever I
said—to think before I spoke.

Once when I was about three years old, I remember hugging
my doll as I climbed the stairs to her bedroom. She was packing a
trunk with her clothes. It was the first time I had ever seen a
trunk. She explained that she would soon be going away from all
of us for a long time with my Grandfather. They would be sailing
on a big ship—a steamship—which would take them around the
world. I felt like crying. I did cry. And then when she was not
looking, I tucked my naked cloth doll with long brown hair like
mine into the corner of her trunk. Ophelia could go with her even
if I couldn't. As weeks passed by I missed my favorite doll.
Gradually, Jocko took Ophelia's place in my arms. My funny,
brown, moth-eaten monkey even slept with me.

My Grandmother's face used to reflect the way she felt when
she looked at my Grandfather. There was an expression in her
eyes and around her mouth—a special sort of smile. Other times
there was a changed tone in her voice—"sarcasm" was the word I
later learned to describe it. She was quick and at times caustic in
her responses—words shot like darts from her tongue.

She often surprised me with her talent for imitating the sounds
of animals or of musical instruments or of the way other people
talked. She was always good-humored and kindly toward me.

Once my Grandmother asked me to help her move some furniture in her guest room. I enjoyed demonstrating my strength.
After the job was done she told me she had something special to
show me. From the dresser's bottom drawer she lifted a large gold
box—a box from China she told me. I was speechless as she
removed the cover and unfolded a length of finely embroidered

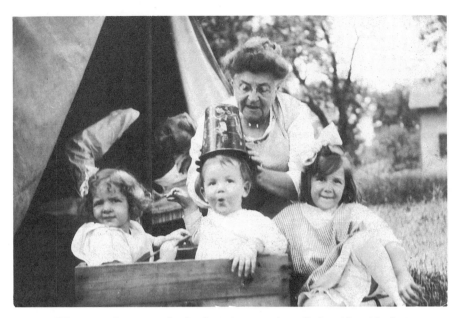

Time together near the backyard tent—three little girls with their grandparents.

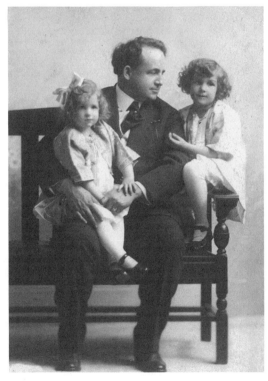

Dressed up in kimonos from Japan.

white silk. With awe I touched its smooth elegance, pressed my fingers over the raised silken thread of the embroidery. "When you grow up this material will be for your wedding dress," she told me as she folded the crepe de chine, replacing it in the gold box.

I was silently ecstatic as I thought, "Grandmother is telling me that some day I shall be married!" Years later when a dressmaker fashioned that same fabric into a beautiful dress for *her*, it was not anger I felt, only a desperate sinking heart. My Grandmother must have changed her mind, was letting me know that she had foreseen my spinsterhood!

My sister Andra and I posed with childish pride the day we dressed in the colorful kimonos our Grandmother had brought home to us from Japan.

She was just over five feet tall, sturdily built. Not in the least obese, her posture erect as she was standing or seated. It seemed to me that her face had always been marked with criss-crossing lines that deepened when she laughed. Her hair had always been gray and she wore a matching hairpiece called a switch, which she twisted and secured with gray hairpins at the top of her head in a neat flattened knot.

Her dresses were long and cottony. Her footgear, unlike my Mother's fashionable high-heeled shoes, were black with laces which tightened as she pulled, and fitted high up over her ankles. Walking was a daily activity for her — usually toward a purposeful destination.

I remember running along beside her, my small hand nested in hers. Often we headed for her flower garden far to the rear of the red brick house. Together we picked flowers — red, yellow, white pink, purple. Back in the kitchen I liked to stand on a stool by the sink as she snipped the stems and arranged them. I can still smell the fresh-cut sweetness and see the old-fashioned gold and white porcelain vase that held them.

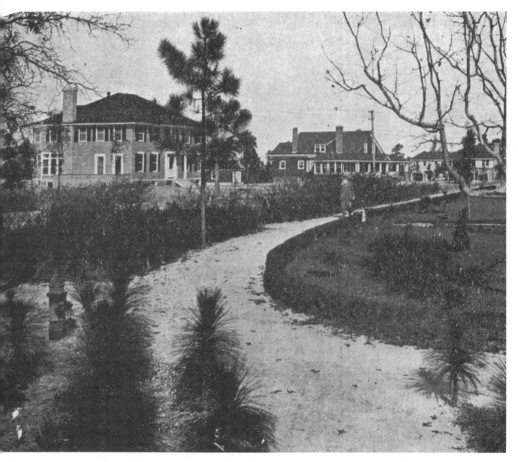

Grandmother's North Carolina bungalow, second house, as it was in 1919.

My Grandmother never cooked—had no interest in kitchen affairs except for directing culinary perfection. The clock preordained the time for meals as daily schedules shifted and Edith performed her special kitchen magic. Edith, German-born, lived with my Grandparents. Endowed with patience, calloused hands, an expanded midriff and flat feet, Edith could do anything. Not only did she cook and manage all the housework, but she doted on my Grandparents. Sometimes for my sisters and me she would sing German songs.

Around the perimeter of the oak paneled dining room stretched a plate rail displaying a parade of china, each telling a separate story. One of them, a brown lava-encrusted plate, had come from the island of Martinique in the Caribbean Sea. Mt. Pelée, a volcano on the island had erupted just a few hours before our Dad had landed on the beach from a small sailboat. Few inhabitants had survived near the still smoking volcano. While exploring a deserted lava-covered street he found the plate crackled and discolored but intact, carried it home as a gift for his Mother.

Hanging over the mahogany dining table, in its unique and threatening way, was a huge gaudy yellow Tiffany glass light fixture. Many years later when it became my inherited task to dismantle my Grandparents' home, it was I who carried that valuable fixture to the curbside to be picked up by trashmen, more experienced and discriminating than I.

My Grandmother not only cheered for rights for women, but she fought for them in her way. Votes for women. Better and equal pay for women. Birth spacing. Better family planning for women. I can remember her parading down East Genesee Street with a host of other black-skirted ladies—drums beating, fifes piping, flags and banners flying. Surprisingly, all the marchers carried eggbeaters with long bright colored streamers labeled "Rights for Women" catching the breezes as the blades twirled. Those eggbeaters symbolized domestic rebellion and changes-to-

come. I cherished her eggbeater for years without precisely under-
standing its significance. Names of other women became familiar.
Carrie Nation, Elizabeth Cady Stanton, Harriet Beecher Stowe,
Susan Anthony, Lucy Stone, Matilda Gage.

One early morning my Grandmother with a tinge of excitement
in her voice called my sisters and me to come to their front porch.
There at our eye level we watched a large spider spinning her
web. We must have stood there enraptured for at least a half
hour. Time seemed not to pass. The sun glinted on the fine silky
threads as the filament expanded and a fly was caught, enmeshed
as he fought desperately to escape. Grandmother talked, as we
watched the fly, about "survival of the fittest."

Another time she called us at dusk to watch a butterfly slowly
emerge from its cocoon — a wonderful sight. After a suitable
period of drying and stretching his wings, the monarch butterfly
fluttered off. The process in its entirety *was* memorably awesome.

One warm summer morning — beautiful for rollerskating — I
fell on the sidewalk in front of our house. Bleeding and crying, I
limped to my Grandmother. After thoroughly washing my knee
with soap and water followed by a stinging alcohol swab she
applied a professional bandage. Speaking conversationally about
the hurtful laceration and about the blood that had been streak-
ing down my leg, she chose that moment to explain to me the
principle of blood circulation. As I stood before her in the
bathroom she pointed out with simple words how my blood was
keeping me alive. My heart was the pump, she said, that continues to beat as long as I would live. It was the same pump that
moved blood through a maze of small tubes from my head to my
toes and back again, being refuelled by oxygen from the air I
breathed into my lungs. With gentle fingers, she traced the cir-
cuit of veins and arteries up and down my arms and legs. In a few

days she assured me, a scab would form over the hurt spot. That would be Nature's way of healing. She had given me the first of many future lessons in physiology.

———————

At home around the dinner table and at school as well, reports about the devastating war in Europe continued. It was April of 1917. Posters were everywhere picturing Uncle Sam wearing his tall red, white and blue hat and pointing his finger at us. Our Grandmother told us that she had lived through three wars involving the United States and now this World War would be the fourth. Enlisted soldiers were already being trained to fight the Germans and were being sent across the ocean on huge liners that were never used before as warships. U-boats, or submarines, were a constant threat. We learned the expression "war casualty" and what it meant.

It wasn't until our good neighbor, Ernest Johnson, appeared at our door in his soldier's khaki uniform that the war hit our lives with reality. It had been Ernest's Friday night treat to drive us all to the drug store at the foot of the hill for chocolate ice cream cones. No more.

There was much talk about the rationing of food and the planting of vegetable gardens, children being "farmerettes." One day when I walked to the grocery store to get our allotment of sugar, the young man at the counter gave me a small sack of salt instead!

At dinner a new ruling demanded that we finish every scrap of food whether we liked it or not. We were told seriously "to remember the starving Armenians." And we saved all our used toothpaste tubes "for the metal to be melted down for bullets." Hard logic for children to comprehend.

Otherwise, World War I seemed not to touch our lives until it ended on November 11, 1918. Then church bells rang, whistles blew, autos blew their horns, school bells tolled as children ran to their homes—laughing and cheering. School closed early!

———————

One day in June 1918

As I walked past the front entrance to the red brick house I caught a glimpse of my Grandmother through the living room window. She was seated in her favorite chair, her attention riveted on the book she was reading. She hadn't seen me as I half-ran past the house that cloudy afternoon.

I had been ringing doorbells in the neighborhood, selling tickets for a benefit movie to be shown the next Saturday afternoon at the Strand Theater. My pile of pink tickets held together with a white rubber band had shrunk to a slim pack. Only seven left as I flipped through them. Sick children at the new hospital would be the beneficiaries.

I had been more than shy and a bit frightened at the prospects of ringing doorbells at strangers' houses. Mother encouraged me by saying that I wasn't asking for anything for myself, but for other children. She handed me a blue leather pouch with change in it so that if anyone might say they didn't have the proper amount right now, I could respond with, "That's all right, I have change right here or I can come back later when your husband comes home." She told me to be sure to smile when a lady came to the door, to introduce myself and to explain that the ticket was for a special movie called "The Bluebird" by a famous man named Maurice Maeterlinck, that it was for grownups and children too and would be shown next Saturday afternoon. All the money would be given to the hospital. She warned me to be polite and say thank you even if I couldn't sell a single ticket. She gave me a hug and sent me on my way.

After I had rung the doorbells on either side of Allen Street I headed home skipping most of the way. On the way I decided to stop at my Grandmother's house to tell her how much money I had collected. She greeted me with a happy tone of voice as I burst into her living room.

She told me she had been collecting money too that very day for the Red Cross. Money was needed for "war work." She explained that it wasn't only money that the Red Cross needed. They needed people to roll bandages, people to knit scarves and sweaters, nurses to help care for wounded soldiers at oversea's hospitals. They needed strong men too to load crates of material onto trains that would later be shipped to France. All these people would be called "volunteers." And, she added, I had been a volunteer too as I rang doorbells for the benefit of children in the hospital right here in our own city.

She then picked up the newspaper she had been reading and pointed to a picture of a group of young women who were caring for undernourished children at a summer camp on a small lake outside the city. As she tapped her finger on the photograph she looked at me and said, "When you grow up you too could be this sort of volunteer. You could tell stories to the children and help in many different ways."

I spoke to my Father that night about what she had told me. A far-away look came into his eyes as he asked me if I ever knew about the terrible fire that had burned her church several years ago. No, nobody had ever told me. "Sit here on the arm of my chair and I shall tell you about another sort of volunteer." It seemed to me that he was sharing a secret with me. "At that time" — his voice was low and deep — "there was great need for the church people to work together for the reconstruction. Luckily, there were members of that church from the university who were not only dedicated to the church and to the minister, but were knowledgeable in architecture. Some of these men were also friends of your Grandfather who talked to him about the plans for reconstruction. Spurred on by your Grandmother's hopes and dreams, he decided to do what he could to help make the beautiful new stone church a reality. Two whole years of hard work.

"Although he seldom occupies the seat next to her in their pew, your Grandmother now considers the University Avenue Church not only her church, but *his* too."

It was one summer day when my Grandfather had driven up north to fish with Nick Peters. My Grandmother asked me to have supper alone with her and sleep overnight in Grandfather's bed.

There was a storm. Thunder, lightning, rain like the tramping of feet on the roof. A flash of lightning flooded the room, reflecting the bolt in the mirror above her dresser. I missed my sisters. I shivered.

Soon my Grandmother came up to the room very quietly, since she must have thought I was asleep. She undressed in the dark, draping her clothes on a chair while I could hear water filling the big tub in the adjoining bathroom.

After her bath, she appeared in her long white nightgown. I watched her in the shadowed room loosen the hairpins that held the hairpiece to the top of her head, watched her as she brushed her hair, watched her as she opened a jar of sweet-smelling cold cream on her dressing table, watched her as she smoothed it onto her face and throat with circular motions, watched her as she screwed the top back onto the jar and rubbed her hands together.

After pulling herself between the linen sheets of her bed, she quietly took out her upper teeth, then her lower teeth and slid them almost silently into a water-filled glass on the little table between the two beds.

I whispered, "Good night, Grandmother."

She reached her hand to my Grandfather's bed. For a long moment we held hands as she said, "I love you, Honney-girl." Even without teeth in place, I could understand her.

My Grandmother went to church regularly. I used to wonder why, because she always complained to my Grandfather about the sermon when she came home. He was a silent listener — a stolid Christian non-churchgoer.

When the weeks of fall rolled around, I remember the smells about their house: the pungent odor of sauerkraut ripening in a barrel down cellar, Edith's ginger cookies baking, the stale smell of my Grandmother's bedroom when she was sick, the late red apples lined up on the porch-step wall, the dried pink rose petals clustered in a lacquered box. I remember the silver coffee pot, the aroma of fresh-brewed coffee at the breakfast table the first time I tasted it. I liked the sweet, creamy, warm flavor of it.

And I learned to tell time from the old great-grandfather clock in my Grandmother's house. It ticked on and on and chimed four times in an hour as it seemed to guard the stair landing where it stood in its corner niche.

When I was nine years old the world seemed to me to have come to an end. In our family, a fifth child was born—a premature tiny brother. And my Mother was dead. DEAD! Haltingly our Father tried to explain to us that Mother was away, that she had gone to Heaven.

Reality for me was that she had completely disappeared, would never be coming back to us again, would never answer my call when I came home from school. The house was empty of her. The grief, beyond tears, which I felt lured me into her dark clothes closet where her dresses still hung, where I could wrap myself in the familiar soft folds. The darkness comforted me. There I could breathe her perfume—not a bottled spray perfume, but the essence of her.

Heaven. Was that somewhere in the sky? I was confused. Death —Heaven. My strong Father's tears, his pale face. Was I an orphan?

I needed my Grandmother. I ran to her house, found her reading. Without a word she stood. With that special smile of hers she greeted me, encircled me in her arms and held me close to her warm-bosomed body until I stopped sobbing. Somehow I felt better, comforted. Often I returned to her warm embrace.

Months after Mother's death, my Grandmother invited me to have supper alone with her in the little breakfast room off their kitchen. We talked about Heaven and Hell and Death. She told

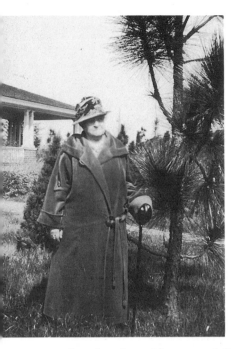
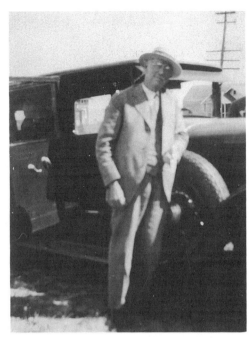

Grandmother with cane and Grandfather with new Franklin car in front of the bungalow.

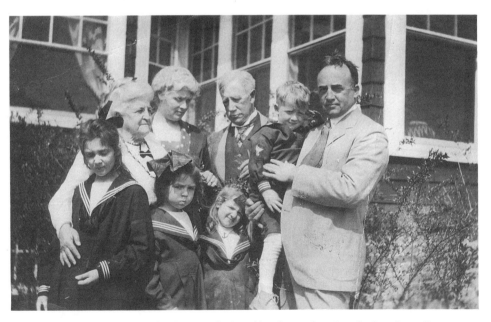

Family photo beside the North Carolina bungalow just before boarding the train for the long trip home in April 1919, one month before Mother's death during childbirth.

me that no person in the world had ever come back to our world from Heaven—or for that matter from Hell—to tell us what it looks like, what it feels like to be there.

She explained that we have been taught that only good people go to Heaven. "That may be true," she continued, "but I am not living my life with the intention of earning a place in Heaven. I am simply living the best I can today and tomorrow and on and on. I am not looking for a reward."

After a long pause as she looked at me with her serious hazel eyes, she placed her hand on mine and said, "I like to think that you are part of me—a part that will go on living a useful life after I die. In a miraculous sort of way, you could be my Heaven." I must have scowled, puzzled. She went on. "As you grow older you will understand that you are part of both your fine parents, your mother and your father. You and your sisters and brothers have been born because they lived and loved together. Each one of you have been given life—have been given a torch wondrously lit by them."

I liked the thought that I was carrying an invisible torch. I wondered if some day I too might be able to pass a lit torch on to a child of my own. The concept of generations was born in my mind.

My deep sorrow bit by bit dispersed. I didn't cry by myself any more. I stopped searching the sky for glimpses of Heaven and my Mother's face in the clouds. I talked with my Father about the small motherless baby still being cared for in the hospital. Would he live? What name would he have? What could we do? Who would take the place of our Mother? The recall of those days still evokes emotion—sharp, painful.

My Mother was thirty years old when I was born, the eldest of five children, all of whom joined the family within the span of ten years. At the premature birth of the last child, my Mother died of a massive hemorrhage, leaving a tiny son whose claim to life was fragile and uncertain.

There had developed scant similarity between the two women

—my Mother and my Grandmother—in the realm of lifestyle and philosophy of child-rearing. Inevitably, contact between the two became increasingly strained in spite of their living next door to each other. My Father, acting more and more in the role of peace-maker, tended inevitably to sympathize with my Mother.

And when my Mother shed tears, so did I.

My Mother as his wife and my Grandmother as his mother, were linked together through passionate closeness to my Father as well as by the fact that only a driveway separated their homes.

Incompatability grew from disparity of their backgrounds. My Grandmother, born and raised on a farm in a loving Presbyterian family contrasted with my Mother's early years as an only child brought up as a Roman Catholic in the city where mother and daughter lived in a third floor apartment. Her father's business as a salesman kept him away from home much of the time. After her graduation from school, Mother found secretarial employment.

My Grandmother's medical education contrasted sharply with that of my Mother's, who had shown early talents as an artist and musician—talents that she pursued throughout her life. Discrepancies in style and physical endowment further separated their ability to understand each other.

Discounting the difference in their ages, the contrast was striking. My Grandmother, short and stocky in stature, was plain in dress, book-loving, quick to make judgments, acerbic in confrontation, imperious in management of her business affairs and in dealing with adversaries. To her ideals and her proven friends, she was loyal and scrupulously devoted.

In stunning contrast, my Mother was unusually tall, blonde, blue-eyed, handsome, fun-loving, energetic and tenderly caring. Compared to my competitive, matter-of-fact, dignified Grandmother, Mother dealt with her family, her peers, household help in a spontaneous, generous, witty and warm-hearted manner.

It was not until after my Mother's death when I was nine years

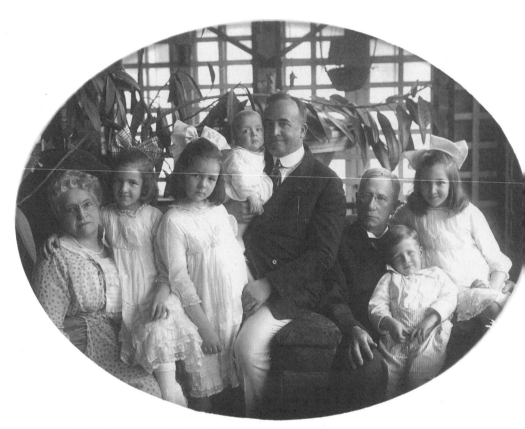

Family group gathered at the time of Baby Donald's christening in the solarium of our house, 1920.

old that my Grandmother's influence on our household became unmistakable. Seldom did she actually come into our house, but the conferences with my Father were daily. She had long been an advocate of "healthful living." The extended family of motherless children were soon to become a living test for validity of her philosophical beliefs.

An open air sleeping porch was constructed at the side of our house. We loved being out there during the summer months. But when the nights became chilly, we were outfitted in Doctor Denton sleepers with built-in feet to keep us warm. We wore knitted helmets and were ensconced all together in sleeping sacs made from old woolen blankets. We slept on that porch until after snow fell. As my Grandmother remarked, "These three girls shall not grow up to be hothouse flowers."

In winter we wore long-legged, long-sleeved woolen underwear, flannel underskirts as petticoats and high-laced shoes. Wool caps, mittens, scarves, heavy coats, leggings and arctics (overshoes) were mandatory. Preparation for going out-of-doors became a hated chore.

It seemed to us that other children at school did not have to dress as we did. Some girls even wore high socks exposing their bare knees in winter!

With Mother no longer at the helm of our household, our Grandmother's influence increased by leaps and bounds. Secretly I didn't welcome the enforced changes.

I attempted in my ten-year-old fashion to take Mother's place myself. I assumed a new voice of authority when I spoke to the younger children. They ignored me. At the end of the day I met my Father at the door when he returned from his downtown office, as Mother had always done. I tried to imitate the way she used to talk to him. I knew the words but didn't understand their meaning. I hugged him.

I sat in her place at the dining room table and at breakfast made the toast. I helped my Father to serve the food. On Saturday nights I shined all our shoes for the next morning's Sunday

School. I told my sisters what to wear. I read stories aloud to the younger children. When they were sick I cleaned up their vomit. The result was that I was miserable. There were inevitable arguments and bouts of hair pulling. Everyone missed Mother and everyone seemed to hate me for trying to impersonate her. Dissention reigned.

Grandmotherly edicts during the second polio epidemic, the summer after our Mother had died, were many. Examples: All children must stay within the confines of the family yard until the danger of disease contagion passed. The cook was told to boil all milk and all water, that only vegetables from Grandfather's garden could be eaten and they should all be cooked thoroughly. There should be no visitors—adult or children—not even my best friend who lived three blocks down the hill.

So it was that Alice and I conspired to locate a secret place by the privet hedge bordering the sidewalk in front of our house to be our mailbox. Under a large stone we hid our private messages to each other—all written in rhymed Morse Code—typical of ten-year-old lyricists.

We read all the Oz books and discussed them at length on a daily basis over the telephone. We were completely immersed in their magic.

There were many other edicts besides isolation. I am sure my Grandmother influenced our Father in the purchase of children's khaki overalls with long sleeves and metal buttons for each one of us to wear for play. A weather eye was kept on us, ever on the alert for signs of fever, vomiting or muscle weakness.

We jumped roped, we climbed trees, we hung by our knees from high branches, we rode our bicycles, we played jackstones with a small rubber ball, we played inventive variations of hide and seek, blind man's buff, hopscotch and marbles, we had ongoing contests at the croquet court. We read books, we played cards and invented plays and games. We learned to embroider.

On rainy days we secretly took off our clothes—especially those heavy overalls—and shook the wet spray from the bushes onto one another. Our nudity did not receive the approval of our scowling Grandmother. She would prefer dowsing us, garbed in bathing suits, with cold water from the hose.

At our Grandmother's house there were many things for children to enjoy—card games to be played, puzzles to be solved, riddles to be devised, hide and seek, blind man's buff, sewing stitches to be learned, more stories to listen to, and Thanksgiving dinners all together.

In an upstairs closet there was what our Grandmother called "a dress-up trunk" filled with old-time finery—male and female cast-offs, hats, shoes, fans, jewelry—even body-covering striped bathing suits.

There were clogs brought from China, Japanese kimonos, Indian shawls, Mexican serapes and all sorts of imaginative stuff. There were even wigs to inspire many a play and charade.

And there was a curving oak bannister to slide down when our Grandmother wasn't looking.

Once there was a Halloween party at our house. Many neighborhood children came outfitted in weird and fanciful costumes.

My Grandmother appeared too as a "paper boy." Through our front door she dashed dressed in a boy's tattered shirt and knee breeches, with a visored cap pulled well down on her head to hide her hair and to disguise her besmirched face. Under one arm she carried a bundle of newspapers as she called "Extry - extry. Read all about it! Extry papah! Git all de noos!" Not one of us recognized her.

On many occasions after supper, our Father supervised neigh-

borhood contests of racing over the front lawn as our Grandparents cheered. "On your mark — Get set — Go!" always with
spatial advantage provided for the younger, shorter-legged children.

When the stars came out, our Father taught us to recognize the
Big and Little Dippers, the Evening Star and the red star of Mars.
He explained to us the various phases of the moon and talked
with us about the "Milky Way" and the aurora borealis.

On Sunday nights in his study he read us O'Henry stories and
poems by Will Carleton. I especially now remember O'Henry's
"The Gift of the Magi" and Will Carleton's poems "The Doctor's
Story" and "Over the Hill to the Poorhouse." We knew them all,
almost by heart. And we talked. Our Father talked to us and we
talked to our Father.

We looked forward to other nights when our Father would
announce it was time to have a "rough house." On those evenings
he would take off his jacket and tie, his shoes and socks, lie down
on the old carpet in the hall and invite us to clamber over him
until he had to call a halt. We played as if we were puppies
scrambling over one another in an effort to be the first to turn
him over. On all "fours" he would then become a "horse" for us to
ride from one end of the long hall to the other.

Finally with appropriate music coming from the old Edison
record player we would pull him to his bare feet and with complete abandon dance until it was bedtime.

As my sisters and I sat in the heat of a sunny August afternoon
with our Grandmother, we were overflowing with questions.

"Grandmother, tell us about the olden days when you were a
little girl. Weren't there any automobiles then? Or any airplanes
either? Did you have ice cream cones then? Did you really have to
go into a separate shed in your backyard to go to the toilet?"

"Grandmother, where did you go to school? Was it really in just
a one-room schoolhouse? Did you have books like we have? Did

you have desks with inkwells and chairs fastened to desks the way we do? Did you have to walk a long way? What did you take in your lunch box? What did the teachers do when boys were bad? Or were girls bad too? What did they do?"

She told us many stories about her growing up on the farm. And always there would be a story that we loved to hear. It was about her wedding in the winter time when she was very young, how she had worn a beautiful white dress with a long train and how flowers were woven into her hair even though it was winter.

And she told us about all the things that had happened to her that year she was married. She moved away from all the people that she knew and loved, away from her father and mother, away from all the farm animals she used to help her father care for, away from her friends and all the little children she used to teach in a small schoolhouse.

She and her new husband went to live far away in a city where her husband worked with five of his six brothers making the kind of sleighs and carriages that were drawn by horses before there were any automobiles or trucks. And in that strange city she had to learn how to cook because her mother had never taught her to bake or make meals for the family when she was growing up.

One time she told us that because people in New England, where they lived, liked to have baked beans for supper on Saturday nights she tried to fix this special favorite supper for her husband. She took down her brown clay pot, mixed the dried beans with molasses and vinegar and salt pork, put them into her oven and cooked them all day. But at supper time the beans were just as hard as when she had placed them there in the morning. She told us she hardly ever cried, but that time she cried. That was how she learned that dried beans must soak overnight before anyone can cook them.

One time she told us the story of how her handsome young husband became desperately sick from a terrible disease known as Typhoid Fever. After only a few days he died. With a faraway look in her eyes, she told us about packing up her belongings including the little maple wood cradle that her husband had carved for their new unborn baby, saying a sad goodbye to all her New Haven family and finally traveling by train to the little town in New York State where her Father and Mother lived. Her baby boy, born on February 7th, grew up to be our Father!

She went on to tell us that in one year many changes influenced the course of her life. She had been a school teacher, a bride, a widow, a mother, a teacher again and a lady who wrote for a newspaper.

The Nineteenth Amendment to the United States Constitution was passed on August 26, 1920 stating that "The rights of citizens of the United States to vote may not be denied or abridged by the U.S. or any State on account of sex. The Congress will have the power to enforce this Article by legislation."

Through a network of telephone communication and coopera- tive action my Grandmother lead a mass invasion of the hall in the neighborhood which had been designated as the Place for Registration. The line-up began to form early in the morning before many men had arrived. And I was among them holding tight onto my Grandmother's hand. She had explained to me that this was an important day—one that I should remember.

One by one the ladies advanced up the stairs of Westminster Hall and into the room where tables had been set up with officials ready to authorize the signatures and addresses of each voter. This, my Grandmother explained, was necessary "registration" prior to allowing each individual to vote on the first Tuesday after the first Monday of November. She spoke on our way home about the importance of this day to every woman in every State of our Union. And she told me not to forget that as soon as I was twenty- one years old I could vote too!

One piece of wonderment in our Grandmother's living room

was the big player piano. I could sit on the long bench beside my Grandmother as she prepared to perform a miracle. Irregularly pierced slits on a yellow music roll fitted into slots and rotated within a small box-like compartment with sliding doors above the keyboard. With a slight movement of her right hand as she shifted an inconspicuous metal lever, my Grandmother performed the miracle that transformed her into a talented pianist. The sound of the "Anvil Chorus" changed the room into a blacksmith shop. Clang-clang reverberated throughout the room. I could practically see the blacksmith and hear his hammer hit a red hot horseshoe. Happy sounds!

There came a day when I could sit alone on that bench, fit a new roll into the box, fix the magic lever to "on," stretch my legs so that my feet could reach the pedals that empowered the keys to dance as the music roll unwound. "Beautiful Ohio in Dreams Again I See, Visions of What Used to Be." My make-believe talented fingers flew over the keyboard!

Next to the piano was a small antique cherry table with two drawers. In the top drawer my Grandmother kept her gloves—the long white kid gloves that she rarely wore and the short white cotton gloves (some without fingers) that she wore when she went for walks or to call on a neighbor. There were brown kid gloves and black ones too, all folded neatly and done up in tissue paper.

In the lower drawer my Grandmother kept her collection of eye glasses. One pair was called a "pince-nez"—frameless, fitted with a gold nose clamp and a loop of black ribbon. When she tried them on she looked like an illustration from one of my story books. There was a magnifying glass monacle with a gold handle and another pair of glasses which when she was not using them, could be retracted to a gold pin attached to the bodice of her dress. There was another pair of steel-rimmed eye glasses with temple pieces to fit around her ears. They were "bifocals" to ease her vision both for close work and distance as well. I tried them all, but the room blurred strangely.

In the same drawer was a tubular box containing "hatpins."

These were long steel pins decorated at one end with a pearl or colored bead, used to secure my Grandmother's hats to her head. She told me that Auntie Johnson always carried an extra hatpin along with her diamond rings in her handbag if she went out alone in the evening — to be used as a weapon in case she were attacked by a strange man!

When I was a little girl I remember sitting beside my Grandmother in a small cane-seated rocking chair I called my own. It was in her living room. She was serving tea to a neighbor — a straight-laced lady with a rasping voice. We heard the door open as my two younger sisters came running into the house. "Twinkle Toes and Little Sister" my Grandmother announced. One, a beautiful blonde, curly-haired child, Andra, older but smaller than four-year-old Franny, who was beautiful too — auburn-haired, brown eyes, chubby and smiling. They both came skipping into the room, curtsied — each in her own fashion — grinned at me and flopped down on the tiger skin rug in front of the fireplace. Soon conversation between the tea-drinking ladies — both honoring the fashion trend of the day by encircling their throats with black velvet bands, became a bore to Andra and Franny who with a secret signal from the older sister made their departure.

As they disappeared into the hallway my Grandmother, using her analytical tone of voice, began to describe the differences between these two grandchildren. "Andra is one of the prettiest little girls I have ever known," she remarked. "Franny too," she continued, "has always been a lovable, cuddly child, but I wonder if she will outgrow those pig-eyes of hers."

Franny, in the hallway, heard her Grandmother's words, "pig-eyes." Never would she forget or forgive that hateful image bestowed on her by her own grandmother. For years whenever she looked skeptically at herself in a mirror she could see eyes from a PIG blinking back at her under her very own quizzical eyebrows!

On various occasions my Grandmother liked to talk to us about the strange and interesting men who visited our neighborhood. She knew instinctively that if she provided a large bowl of ripe red apples as we sat cross-legged on the floor near her, we would forget that time was passing as we listened to her stories.

One day she asked us if we had noticed a big chalk mark in the form of an X on the sidewalk in front of her house. Of course we had. We thought it was left by boys playing some sort of game.

That X is a secret symbol she told us. "It's a sign put there by a 'hobo' who has been here before. He knows this house. He has provided a signal to any of his hobo friends who may come this way that here is a place where they can all be given food. 'Hoboes' or tramps as they are sometimes called, are men without jobs who hop freight trains, travel in box cars inside or on top, from city to city, town to town. Hoboes league themselves into bands. When they land in an area they like, they jump off the trains and go out singly from the railroad yards in search of food or money. The X on the sidewalk means 'welcome to be found here.' Your Grandfather and I always give them food, but never money. They usually want money for whiskey." She told us it was all right to talk with them even if they were dirty and smelly, but never to let them come into the house — never to let them touch us.

There was another sort of man who used to come by her house. He was "the hurdy-gurdy man," always appearing with his "organ grinder" and his little monkey dressed in bright colored coat and pants, with a hole in the rear for his tail. While his master played the tiny hand organ, the monkey danced at the end of a chain to the tunes the organ played and then took off his red feathered cap and passed it to gather pennies from the cheering children. We always loved the Hurdy-Gurdy Man.

On certain days of the week during the summer and fall, the Huckster Man with his old horse and wagon, would clop-clop into the driveway, calling in a sing-song Italian vernacular, "Fresh tomatoes, potatoes, corn and beans, crispy cucumbers. Bananas, pineapples, extra big oranges!" Neighbors gathered to deal with

him as he measured his produce into tin containers or onto his
rickety scales produced from the dark corner of his wagon. My
Grandmother warned him about driving carefully as he turned
into our yard. But special joy came to us when he lifted the neighborhood children two by two, onto the seat beside him as he sang
Italian ditties and drove his horse around the circle of our
driveway.

There were other days when we looked forward to giving our
knives and scissors to the "Sharpening Man" who announced his
coming by calling in a loud voice, "Dull knives to sharpen — Old
scissors to grind — Worn-out tools to make new! Come one, come
all." He carried his honing wheel strapped with leather thongs to
his shoulder. We stood in awe at the flying sparks as his pedal-
powered wheel spun around and around. Sometimes our Grandmother would give us money to pay him and let us take dulled
scissors to him to sharpen.

And then there was the Rag Man with his bony mule and
ancient cart. He would call, "Old rags — Old papers — Old rags —
Old papers — I'll buy your old rags!" We wondered what he did
with them. Our Grandmother told us.

And the Bee Man who came to Grandmother's door with boxes
of honey-in-the-comb, a sweet waxy miracle. Many times she
repeated the story of the bees and the flowers and the unique
royalty of the hives.

There were other days when gypsy bands passed her house
riding in a parade of horse-drawn carts, painted in bright colors.
"Watch out for them, children," she warned us. "Sometimes gypsies steal little boys and girls even as they are playing in their own
yards. Go into the house whenever you see them coming."

The warning only increased our wonder. We thought about
how it would feel to be carried to their encampments as in our
imaginations we were tempted to allow ourselves to be carried
away to live in tents with these brightly garbed, tambourine-
shaking, black-haired, dark-skinned, singing gypsies.

At intervals during the year coal was delivered to the cellar of our house. As children we were fascinated with the arrangement of a metal shoot leading from the coal wagon through a designated window to the dark sooty coal bin in our cellar. As the coal began its descent it sounded like a huge waterfall, constant in its turbulance. The men's faces as they guided the delivery looked alike — blackened, unsmiling, bored. They never talked with us.

And there was the Ice Man. He could know by the position of a yellow diamond-shaped card place in the window of her living room how many pounds of ice were needed. The pounds, 25, 50, 75 or 100, were noted in each corner of the card and the top corner gave him the information he needed. He would then hoist the big frozen block of ice onto his rubber-covered shoulder with a pair of huge tongs, carry the ice from his rig at the street curb to the open back door and deposit it inside the big wooden ice box in the kitchen. He always smiled and had a teasing word to say to all of us. Sometimes he let us suck on a piece of chiseled ice.

And then there was the Postman, Walter, who walked miles from house to house in the neighborhood delivering mail once every morning and once every afternoon. His big leather bag was heavy and bulky, but it never seemed too much weight for him to manage. Sometimes he came into the kitchen to have a cup of coffee or glass of lemonade and to tell us about a vicious dog he had made friends with or a lost child he had returned to his worried mother. He was our special friend, but he never came on Sunday.

I remember going with my Grandmother one fine summer afternoon to attend a meeting of the KaNaTeNah Club downtown in Syracuse. A group of literary ladies dressed in Sunday finery, met in a large darkened room of the Hamilton White House overlooking a park. I sat next to my Grandmother while a high-voiced reader spoke for a long time about the rivers in our country. I was very sleepy. My eyes kept closing. I must have been about eight years old.

Another time in September ladies and men too came to my
Grandparents' house for an evening meeting. "Current Events
Discussion" she explained to me. My sisters and I took great
pleasure in watching the people as they arrived at the front door
of the Big Red Brick House.

Another day Grandfather was playing his favorite game of
solitaire. I stood at his side looking over his shoulder. He knew I
was waiting to catch him cheating. Cheating himself of course,
but nevertheless cheating.

It was a hot afternoon in July 1920. His sleeves were rolled up.
He had been working in his garden hoeing the long rows of vege-
tables. He smelled sweaty. Nice sweaty. His face was shiny red.
He was at the card table in his den.

As I looked down at his bony hand poised over the cards, the
blue veins marked a familiar pattern — like a road map. A design
of major and minor blue lanes lead from his sinewy hand up
along his arm to the folded sleeve. A forest of white hairs on his
arm seemed to my squinting eyes to look like tiny bare-branched
trees sprinkled with silver. Still no move as he studied the cards.

My Grandfather was a good farmer. His arms were stong —
especially his right arm. He planted seeds in the springtime, hoed
the hills, tended and fertilized the plants, pulled the weeds,
gathered the vegetables in the fall, picked the berries, stripped
the corn, shared them all with us. And it was this same warm arm
I felt when it encircled my shoulders as I walked with him from
the strawberry patch to meet my Grandmother up by the house
where she was working in her flower garden.

Recovering from my reverie, I watched him maneuver his
cards. I caught him red-handed. He was pulling the black ten of
clubs from the bottom of his pack to place on the waiting jack of
hearts. Cheating again! With a soft chuckle, he winked at me.
How I adored him!

My memory concerning the statuary in the stairway of my Grandparents' house is still clear. It stood probably three feet tall, carved from white marble, transported from Greece to the wide windowsill on the stair landing between the first and second floors of their home. Her robe, draped from one shoulder, hung in graceful folds to her sandalled feet. In spite of having been carved from marble, the material covering her body with utmost modesty, looked soft and loose-fitting.

My Grandmother told us that this kind appearing marble lady represented a Greek goddess, the Goddess of Health, "Hygeia." According to mythology she was a daughter of Aescalapius, God of Medicine. She worked with her father for the good of the people, for those who were well and those who were sick. The serpent with spread eagle wings signified protection, healing and relief from pain.

After death had claimed both my Grandparents, one of my unenviable tasks was to decide what to do with Hygeia. Ultimately the marble statue was carried to the curbside in front of their house—her last commission being to guard the several trash barrels placed there. Knowing trash collectors as I do, I was sure that after losing her head, being disfigured and unrecognizable, Hygeia would end up as a pile of marble rubble and dust in the city dump. I felt no regrets.

At the big red brick house I was searching for Dinah, Grandmother's jet black cat. We knew that she was about to have kittens. She was nowhere to be found downstairs, so I climbed the circling staircase with its oak bannister, past the great-great-grandfather's clock standing in the corner of the landing, glanced up at the marble face of the Goddess Hygeia, tall on her pedestal by the window, and ran up the remaining steps to the second floor. No sign of Dinah until I entered my Grandparents' bedroom. It was then that I heard Dinah meowing—discovered her under my Grandmother's four-posted mahogany bed. I managed

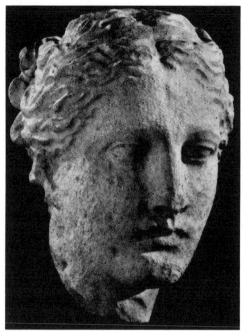

Statue of Hygeia

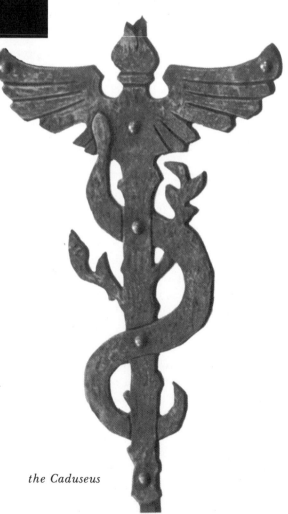

the Caduseus

to gather her into my arms and carried her to her own basket-bed in the garage.

A few days later while I was embroidering a sampler on the porch with my Grandmother, Dinah appeared carrying one tiny black kitten. She held it by the scruff of its neck between her teeth. Forthwith she carefully dropped her tiny baby at my Grandmother's feet and returned to the garage. Four times she returned to the porch, each time carrying another kitten of varying white, brown and black color demarkation to deposit with the others.

They were beautiful but I was concerned that Dinah might have hurt her babies by carrying them grasped between her upper and lower jaws apparently biting the furry skin at the back of their little necks. None of them could even walk yet. They just tumbled over one another making funny kitteny noises. I sat on the floor and stroked them for a little while before Dinah decided it was time to go back to their nest in the garage.

I followed and watched her as she nursed them all—five of them at the same time. I never knew that could happen. And then she licked them clean with her rough pink tongue as they nestled up to her and slept. Dinah purred and soon slept, too.

One winter afternoon we were all sitting on the floor of our Grandmother's den drawing pictures. She took down a small American flag that had been stuck into a framed picture hanging on the wall, a picture of the Capitol building in Washington. She told us that the flag had changed since she was a little girl. The flag then had twenty-nine white stars on it instead of forty-eight. She explained to us that the 29 stars represented 29 states. That's all there were when she was born. She asked us to tell her the difference between 29 and 48. She never forgot she had been a teacher. We asked her about the red and white stripes.

She then told us the story of Betsy Ross and showed us a picture of her as she was cutting out thirteen five-pointed stars and arranging them in a circle on a flag to represent the first thirteen original colonies in America. That happened in her Philadelphia upholstery shop where she had hand-sewn the first flag for our country. My Grandmother then taught us to draw and color that flag as it used to be with its circle of stars and the one now that we salute every day in school with its thirteen red and white stripes and its 48 white stars on a field of blue. She asked us what we thought the colors meant. We talked about red symbolizing blood, blue being truth, and white being purity.

We all loved the stories our Grandmother told us.

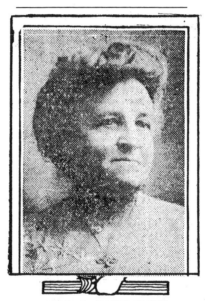

MRS. A. J. DE MOTT
(Hostess at meeting of Syracuse University Alumnae Club.)

One afternoon there was a fancy tea party in the red brick house—a special occasion when our Grandmother was entertaining a large group of ladies from the University, "because she was President of the Alumnae Association." My two sisters and I sneaked up the back stairs from the kitchen in the big house, tip-toed into the bedroom where the ladies had left their hats, gloves, purses and wraps. It was hilarious fun for us to try on the befeathered and beflowered hats—one after the other—and to pose in front of the tall gilt-framed peer mirror as if we had a perfect right to be there. We strutted, we made faces, we giggled. And because there was a serious meeting going on downstairs, no one disturbed us—not even Edith who was too busy in the kitchen to investigate the goings-on in the guest room.

"Where did you get this tiger skin from?" I broke the voice silence in my Grandparents' living room as I stroked the silky head of the fierce looking animal stretched out in front of the fireplace where sparks were sputtering. Grandmother was plucking the strings of her guitar in an attempt to tune it. Grandfather sat at a table by the window, flipping his dog-eared cards as he laid out another triangular pattern for a game of solitaire. It was a Sunday afternoon during the winter of 1922.

"I remember the day clearly," he answered. "I knew even then that your Grandmother would come back home with some cock and bull story about how we had been trudging through the high-lands of India, had been attacked by this tiger dashing from behind a rock. She would like to tell about how brave our guide was and how we watched the beast stumble and fall from the first blast of his gun.

"But really, Honney, that's not the way we got this tiger rug. I'll tell you what actually happened."

My Grandmother continued by interrupting the old man she loved. "One day when we were in Bombay, your Grandfather and I were walking slowly through the market place. It was hot. Native men and women with all sorts of merchandise were hawking their wares, from brass and copper utensils to trays, coffee urns—even tall oil lamps. Each vendor had a cubicle where he stood guarding his treasures. The cubicles were open to the cinder pathway lining the walk on either side of a stinking open sewer. There were other shops where cheap clothing, tablecloths, perfumes and trinkets set with shiny colored glass were sold. There were handwoven rugs and animal skins exhibited on tables and hung on lines strung in front of the shops. Yes, there was one full-grown tiger skin nailed to the wall. We noticed that he had a special glint in his eye. We stared at him, liked his harmless appearance and decided he would be a fine playmate for you children." And she went on, "He was probably not killed with a gun. He was likely trapped."

"What else did you do while you were in India?" I asked. "Well, Honney, I can tell you about a young woman I met on that same alleyway. She wasn't even as tall as you are—thin as she could be and carrying a tiny baby in a sling on her back. The place smelled because of the open sewer ditch running between the walkway and the stalls.

"Flies were everywhere. The baby's head was lolling on the mother's shoulder as I passed and flies were crawling on the newborn's face—one lit on his open eye. Instinctively I brushed my hand over the child's head as I passed. As I did so, the mother looked at me with horror, uttered a curse and tried to slap me on my face. You see, in India no living thing—including flies—should be killed. Their religion has strict taboos. Of course, because I am a doctor I suppose, I was thinking of the fly causing an eye infection—perhaps death to that baby. There is much blindness among the people who live in India." I could understand that she couldn't help thinking like a doctor.

"Well, dear," she went on, "some day there will be Indian doctors who will know the causes for so much blindness among their people and will do something about it. Who knows when that will be. Perhaps by the time you are grown up." She went on to tell about the beauty of the countryside, the mountains, the rain forests where orchids grow.

She then showed me a picture of themselves and a family that they had visited on the island of Ceylon. They were having what they called "high tea," a rather elegant way of serving afternoon refreshments to guests.

She also told me about some of the less elegant customs, such as the burning of the dead. And that among certain religious sects if a husband dies, his wife is expected to die as well, by hurling herself on the funeral pyre.

Her stories were always true stories in spite of Grandfather's fanciful interjections.

———————

I stood alone at the doorway of the den in my grandparents' old red brick house. I was waiting for their return. They had taken their new open touring car to drive along the back country roads to catch a glimpse of the wondrous fall colors just beginning to show in the fields and the woods. That was during the fall of 1925.

Their den, always warm and welcoming to me, took on a different aspect that day. No one was there. I was looking at pictures hung on the wall that I had never really seen before. They were familiar but extraneous, like signposts never before read.

The pictures told the story of their many travels to foreign countries, countries I had never visited except in books. There seemed to be no logical reason for the way the pictures were hung —no continuity of subject matter, no artistic arrangement. The first framed photograph to catch my eye was one of a posed group of people dressed in old-fashioned garb standing at the base of a huge pyramid. There they were, my two grandparents in Egypt. Probably the people with them were their companions from the ship that had taken them around the world.

And there was a bull fight postiviely "at the moment of truth." I remembered some of the costumes they had brought home from Spain. Next to that gory sight was a gilt-framed portrait of an old man, his face weather-beaten, wrinkled and swarthy. On his head was a rust-colored baggy cap flopped over to the side of his face and covering most of his gray hair. His blue eyes stared back at

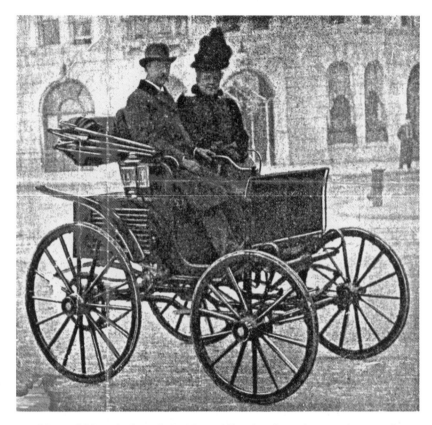

Mr. and Mrs. Andrew J. DeMott riding in a horseless carriage, early 1900s Stanley Steamer.

me—blue like his jacket that was buttoned so that only a flash of white shirt and red scarf showed at his throat. He appeared at extraordinary ease as he smoked his long-stemmed pipe—a flicker of flame in the bowl. I wondered where he had come from. Was he a French Huguenot like my Grandfather?

Behind the card table where my Grandfather played solitaire for hours was a recent group picture of the whole family, each one unsmiling. And near it a series of prints depicting in detail the bloody outcome of a Mexican cockfight from start to gloating dead finish.

On another wall the portrait of a mysterious lady stared out at me from behind her black veils. Beside her and higher on the wall was a picture of the Roman Colliseum. At least I recognized the scene. And further down was a black-framed photograph of both grandparents in a horseless carriage, obviously driving down a main city thoroughfare. What astounded me more than the lack of a horse was the high feathered hat my grandmother was wearing.

On the mantel above the fireplace was a gleaming white marble miniature model of the Taj Mahal and nearby on the same mantel a carved ebony water buffalo with a small Oriental boy astride his neck.

Displayed on the high-backed desk was a replica of a Japanese jinrikisha with wheels that moved. And a Japanese teapot. And a blue cloissonné vase.

I heard the side door click open and close as two of my favorite people in the world came in, ruddy from their windy ride. Laughing, I told them I had been enjoying myself inspecting pictures and memorabilia.

From the bookcase my Grandmother pulled out a scrapbook she had organized, thumbed through its pages as she told me stories about that trip around the world with the steamer trunk in which I had tucked my naked doll, Ophelia, all those many years ago. We talked until the clock struck, about their travels, about funny things that had happened aboard a ship or a camel and about how they had enjoyed hanging a picture here and there in their home to remind them of their adventures. Before I left them, my Grandmother reached high on the wall to remove a carved wooden plate with a scene of Swiss mountains painted on it. With a twist of a key on its underside, the hidden music box played "Der Edelweiss," a tune honoring the tiny white flower that grows on the cliffs in the high peaks of the Alps. The plate she gave me to keep. Over the years I have treasured that gift.

———————————————

As school and then college necessitated separation from home and Grandparents, I was conscious of missing the special banter and human warmth that prevailed under the roof of that red brick house. Appreciation of the close bonding with my Grandmother persisted throughout the years. And the old grandfather clock has ticked on.

I remember the house — its Georgian Colonial architecture, the plantings around it, the trees — their shade in summertime, the falling leaves in autumn, the snow gathering on bare twigs in winter, the pale green budding in spring. Inside that house, with flashes of recognition, I can see the arrangement of furniture in the rooms, the colors, the feel of the fabrics, the pictures on the wall, the artifacts, the row on row of books. I can still smell the books. And I can feel again the safe comfort, the undemanding sense of belonging that surrounded me in that red brick house.

CONTINUUM

CONTINUUM

The following letter, destined never to be answered, suggested the unremitting continuity of one woman's long life. The envelope, torn open, lay amid medicine bottles on the marble-topped table beside her bed. Surely Millie, M.D. had been reading the words on Christmas morning, the final day of her eighty-one years of life.

At Home
December 22, 1927

Dear Grandmother DeMott,

The snow-covered red brick house across the driveway is dark. As I write to you in Dad's study surrounded by his books, I hear the ticking of your old grandfather clock as the hands move toward midnight. It stands now in the corner of this room — its sound and sight comforting to me. Even so I wish I could be near you, to talk with you tonight at this Christmas season.

I hope that the pain around your heart has subsided now that you have left his north country of snow and cold. I like to think of you taking your daily walks under warm, sunny skies — listening to the taunting call of mocking birds and the whistle of cardinals as they fly from holly tree to cedar tree and back again.

I am reminded of the winter not so long ago when our whole family came to stay with you and Grandfather — all of us together under the roof of the brown shingled bungalow. Amazing that we all fitted in!

Both of you, Mother and Dad, the four of us children and
Edith! I wonder now how Edith managed to create three meals
a day on the big black wood stove in the kitchen. How hungry
we all were! I remember well the oval table in the dining room
where Grandfather did all the carving and serving while you
tried to get us all to talk "One-At-A-Time, if you please!" I
remember the first faint music from the then new radio broad-
casting station KDKA in Pittsburgh. And will you ever forget
the clicking scratched records we played over and over again on
the ancient phonograph? And the visits to the deer park! Once I
watched a peacock fall over dead after I had fed him an un-
shucked peanut. I never told you about that—or anyone else.

Riding with Grandfather in the open touring car was a
special treat for us when we headed for a picnic at "the end of
the world" where the red clay road merged with the grassy river
bank.

How we loved to watch the turkey buzzards as they circled
and swooped above us. Best of all I can still smell the spice of a
southern Spring!

The old clock is still ticking—suddenly louder—time for me
to tell you of the incredible dilemma I face. —Your influence
on me over the years may be responsible, my dear Grandmother.

You see, I want to go to medical school—I want to become a
doctor. So far my college experience leads me to further study.
The Dean has encouraged me and with an unmistakable glint
in his eye he says that being a woman should not deter me.

Dad urges me to "Go for it, Daughter. Nothing would make
your Grandmother happier." I wonder. So it is that one of the
paths at the Crossroads leads to the study of medicine and
many more years of dedicated work.

Another path leads back to the house where I grew up. You
have looked me in the eye on several occasions saying,
"Honney, you realize, don't you, that your Father is going to
need you at home when you finish college. He will need you to
run that big house, he will need you to help him as your
younger brothers and sisters grow up—each with special problems. When it comes to entertaining his friends your Father is

going to need you—really needs you now." When I realize how serious you were, I have qualms of conscience. I feel guilty.

You know that I love Father deeply—enormously. He has never voiced a wish for me to come back home "to look after him," but from what you have said to me, the idea must be a hope in the back of his mind.

Well, the third path leads me directly toward marriage. You must believe that I am heart and soul in love. Who is he? He is honest, intelligent, tall, dark, handsome—a man finely attuned to living life to its fullest. I want you to meet him. The sensation I now feel is different from any other I have ever experienced. At one moment I am flying in ecstasy—the next I'm dissolving in tears. He senses the ebb and flow of my emotions as we talk together about marriage, about children— your great-grandchildren—about the joining and focusing of our separate lives.

And yet—and yet—I am totally conscious of needing to BECOME—to become more than love alone may empower.

Clearly I can hear you say as many other times before tonight you have said to me, "Of course, my dear—but you know the decision must be yours alone—yours and only yours."

The old clock is just now striking one o'clock. And in the morning with my Christmas love tucked in, this special delivery letter begins its long, winding train ride to you.

Honney

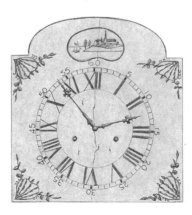